@beautysi

THRIVE STATE

SECOND EDITION

YOUR BLUEPRINT FOR OPTIMAL HEALTH, LONGEVITY, AND PEAK PERFORMANCE

klen@bienvuumd.com
626 673 5436

KIEN VUU, MD

@doctorvmd.

Published by Kien Vuu, MD
kienvuu.com

ISBN 978-1-949680-45-4 (paperback)
ISBN 978-1-949680-46-1 (ebook)

Printed in the USA

Get resources and connect with me.

PRAISE FOR *THRIVE STATE*

"Open, honest, scientifically-backed health information from a physician who walks his talk. *Thrive State* provides a step-by-step guide to longevity and peak performance that anyone can utilize to live their best life."

~ Shawn Stevenson
Bestselling author of *Sleep Smarter* and *Eat Smarter*

"Dr. Vuu really knows his stuff. *Thrive State* is actionable and full of useful health information. If you want to be fully inspired and laugh while learning, he's your guy!"

~ Dave Asprey
Father of Biohacking and 4x New York Times Best Selling Author

"*Thrive State* reminds us that, ultimately, health and performance is not just about the emerging technologies in medicine, but the art of how we live our lives. Dr. Vuu blends intuition and spirituality with the science of longevity; *Thrive State* is truly a gem for the soul."

~ Serena Poon CN, CHC, CHN
Celebrity Chef & Nutritionist

"The Fountain of Youth is at our fingertips and Doctor V is handing you the key. Doctor V has spent his career on the forefront of anti-aging unlocking the door between new discoveries and technologies and your body's ability to harmonize with them. In *Thrive State*, Doctor V reveals how you can unlock that power to achieve optimal health and performance while loving the process."

~ George Bryant
New York Times bestselling author of *The Paleo Kitchen*

"A must read. *Thrive State* is an empowering framework that reminds us We Are Our Best Medicine."

~ Keith Ferrazi
2x New York Times bestselling author and Global Thought Leader

"The vision of *Thrive State* is a compelling moonshot with principles that can aid in the eradication of chronic disease and elevation of health consciousness."

~ Naveen Jain
Iconic Entrepreneur and CEO of Viome and Moon Express

"Dr. Vuu has done an excellent job leveraging science and medicine into a 360 degree approach to longevity and performance. His use of personal stories makes this information accessible to individuals or organizations looking to uplevel where they are in life."

~ Jason Wachob,
Founder & Co-CEO, mindbodygreen

"We all know health and performance are important but we get stuck on what to prioritize and why. Doctor V demystifies the confusion and provides a truly executable plan for any individual and organization to Thrive. Doctor V's energy and passion to uplevel human and organizational health and performance are contagious. Side effects may include peak levels of joy, productivity, and resilience."

~ Chris Barton
Founder of Shazam & Innovation Thought Leader

"If you're looking to take your organizational health to the next level, there's nobody better than Doctor V and his *Thrive State* message. He elegantly blends medicine with performance and organizational health to optimize performance and achieve the impossible. Highly recommend his work."

~ Josh Linkner
Innovation Keynote Speaker and 2X NYT Best-Selling Author

"*Thrive State* is full of stories from the heart while weaving in lessons of leading through change, performance intelligence, and mental and emotional resilience. Our members including leaders and executives from music, arts, technology, to businesses of all industries were captivated with his message; *Thrive State* is a true masterpiece."

~ Ken Rutkowski
CBS Radio and Founder of METAL International

"Walking into a crowded room with Dr. V is like opening up a bottle of champagne and passing out full glasses; His sheer charm and unbridled enthusiasm intoxicates anyone in the vicinity. Fully armed with medical expertise but coupled with a true desire to change the world, this guy is the real deal!"

~ Eric the Trainer Fleischman
Hollywood Physique Expert

"In a confusing and conflicting world of medicine, *Thrive State* presents a practical roadmap to health and performance that interlaces science with the physical, mental, emotional, and spiritual dimensions of wellness."

~ Brendan Kane
Best Selling Author of One Million Followers

"Fasten your seat belts because Doctor V will put you back in the driver's seat of optimal health and performance. *Thrive State* is a simple, yet elegant framework that unlocks the medicine and healing powers within ourselves."

~ AJ Buckley
Actor and Star of CBS's *Seal Team* & *CSI New York*

"*Thrive State* is the secret weapon to unleash energy, vitality, and impact in life and business."

~ Ryan Pineda
Iconic Entrepreneur and Content Creator & Former MLB Player

"The Tony Robbins of health! Doctor V is truly an incredible individual with a gift to motivate others to better health."

~ Dr Daryl Blackwell
CEO, Axyon Consulting

"His message of *Thrive State* is rippling positivity, possibility, and empowerment in lives and corporations throughout the world."

~ Daniel Hennes
CEO Engage Speakers Bureau

"Dr Vuu has a masterful way of blending science, medicine, and storytelling to approach change and stress. I'm not only empowered and inspired by his message, but now have the tools to access more resilience, vitality, and productivity."

~ Dan Chuparkoff
Product Leader at Google and alum at McKinsey & Co

"Bringing the framework of *Thrive State* to leadership and leading high performance teams is a game-changer. The book doesn't only present the science behind high performance, but also provides concrete strategies for maximizing our teams emotional health and productivity."

~ Bruce Cardenas
Former Chief Communications Officer at Quest Nutrition

"*All I can say is WOW! . . . Thrive State*'s IMPACT process will help unleash any person's or organization's ability to discover the best versions of themselves—allowing them not only to have a happier healthier life, but have the energy and vitality to fulfill their mission and purpose."

~ Josh Berman
Managing Partner, Troy Capital Partners

For My Parents, for their unconditional love and support.
For Tiffany, who has challenged me to find a higher perspective
and a better version of myself each day. For Kira and Kaia,
who have been my greatest teachers of life and love.

And a very heartfelt thank you to Eric "the Trainer" Fleishman,
whose belief in me inspired me to find my Thrive State
and whose life was the ultimate example of generosity
and service to others.
Your brilliant light will forever live in my heart.

CONTENTS

PREFACE TO THE 2ND EDITION xi

INTRODUCTION: Health & Extraordinary Human Performance
Is in Our DNA. 1

CHAPTER 1: How I Reversed My Chronic Diseases. 7

CHAPTER 2: The BioEnergetic Model & 7 BioEnergetic Elements. 21

CHAPTER 3: Sleeping for Success 39

CHAPTER 4: What the F*#% Should I Eat?. 61

CHAPTER 5: Your Personal Food Blueprint. 83

CHAPTER 6: Getting Your Move On. 111

CHAPTER 7: Mastering Stress, Harnessing Your Emotions 141

CHAPTER 8: Mindset Is Everything 171

CHAPTER 9: Enhancing the Relationships that Enhance You. 197

CHAPTER 10: Rediscovering Your Spirit and Purpose. 219

CHAPTER 11: The Thrive State Advantage: Going From Me To We. . 233

CHAPTER 12: Creating Lasting IMPACT 251

CONCLUSION: YOU Are Your Best Medicine 261

EPILOGUE: Strengthening Your Path Forward. 273

PREFACE TO THE 2ND EDITION

Since the original publication of the first edition of Thrive State in early 2021, I have seen many advances in the field of human performance and longevity. I've also had a chance to witness firsthand the effects of the COVID-19 pandemic in the hospitals, my concierge practice, our communities, and our organizations and businesses. It seems every so often, some outside force—or pressure—will challenge the fabric of an ecosystem. That ecosystem could be the harmony of the many different cells and microbes that make up the human body, or the collective of individuals that work together in communities and teams that form businesses, organizations, and humanity.

There was one common pressure—a virus—yet the aftermath for individuals and organizations couldn't look more different. I've seen many people pass away in the ICU due the complications of COVID pneumonia and others with lingering symptoms of long haul COVID. I've seen families and communities torn apart over health mandates, lockdowns, and forced social distancing. I've seen many businesses and organizations shut down permanently, and others struggling to find workers or support their already mentally and emotionally burdened workforce.

Surprisingly, in the midst of the same pressure, I've seen individuals who were infected by the virus who experienced very mild, short-lived symptoms and no long-term complications, including my entire family and concierge practice. I've also witnessed teams, families, and communities become even stronger and tighter in the midst of pressure. Their connection, support, and love for one another grew from this adversity. Finally, I've seen some businesses absolutely thrive during this pressure, and they seem to be magnets for the best talent no matter what the season.

Why is this?

In combining my entire body of research studying the world's highest performing individuals, longest-lived populations, the most resilient ecosystems (biological, communities, and organizational) with the observations I made over the past few years, I've concluded that there is one overarching trait that seems to distinguish between the humans, communities, and organizations that thrive and get stronger with pressure versus those that don't.

Cells form tissues which form organs which form biological systems which work together to make us who we are. Extraordinary human potential (performance) is the result of the optimization of these systems. This includes: an optimized immune system to protect us against pathogens; an optimized nervous system that allows us to create, innovate, and respond quickly; and an optimized cardiovascular and musculoskeletal system that allows us to scale Mt. Everest, run marathons, and surf giant waves.

Similarly, as individuals, we are merely cells in the larger ecosystem of our families, teams, organizations, and humanity. And in order for the latter to grow, evolve, and thrive, each individual must as well.

It is this observation that prompted me to release this updated, second edition of Thrive State. The Thrive State is the energetic state of being that activates the biology of human potential—health, longevity, and performance. In this new edition, I talk about some of the new and exciting advances in the human performance and longevity space— new diagnostics that facilitate the early detection of disease and changes in physiology. Critically, I also discuss how the Thrive State not only optimizes us as individuals, but how this energetic field we create within ourselves permeates outward, and governs all the ecosystems we are a part of—our families, our communities, and our businesses. Furthermore, I discuss the single most important factor that prevents us from reaching our potential—the Default Mode Network—a primitive aspect of our consciousness and nervous system that has allowed us to survive, but certainly has prevented us from thriving. And, I share a simple IMPACT framework to overcome whatever holds us back from being the best version of ourselves.

After publishing the previous edition, one of my mentors, Tony Robbins, released the book *Lifeforce* with co-authors Peter Diamandis and my friend Dr. Robert Hariri. It's one of the most comprehensive summaries of all the diagnostics, science, medicines, and treatments in the longevity space. It's a great collection of what I call the Science of Longevity. But I wonder how many of us are forgetting about another powerful medicine—the Art of Living?

A paradox exists in the practice of longevity medicine. Our ever-increasing scientific knowledge and technology has allowed us to expand the human lifespan further than ever thought possible. Yet as technology expands, we face significant problems. We have created a world of paradox. We make tall buildings, but we live in them with short tempers. Our view of the world is made wider by the internet, yet our viewpoints seem to be narrower. We are materially richer than ever, yet face a pandemic of sadness and anxiety. All our 'conveniences' seem to give us no more time. As a doctor, I see how we have added more technology and capability to the American healthcare system, yet collectively we are sicker. For all our advances, our lives in many ways are not better. Sometimes I think of a Benjamin Franklin quote:, "Some people die at the age of 25 but are not buried until 75!" With all this science and technology, are we merely pushing back the time we are buried, especially if we forget about CHOOSING to create a beautiful life?

I've studied some of the world's longest-lived populations, and I've learned that they were able to activate the biology of longevity and human performance through conscious choices. And it's through these conscious choices that we activate the Thrive State. With the advent of all these new technologies, we are not fated to simply extend lifespan without expanding, enjoying, or enriching life itself. We can choose our Thrive State.

It is my sincere hope that this book will inspire and empower you to realize the power you have within you to not only achieve optimal health and performance, but to radiate your gifts to others so that your families, your organizations, and the world can become the best version of themselves as well. Thank you for investing your time and attention with this book; I know that as you start to implement the suggestions I put forth, you'll begin to unlock new possibilities within yourself and the planet.

HEALTH & EXTRAORDINARY HUMAN PERFORMANCE IS IN OUR DNA

D o you want the good news or the bad news first?

This is a question I've asked hundreds of my patients over the years, from those struggling with life-threatening diseases to those who've come into my concierge practice for medical advice on how to take their health and performance to the next level. Often, the good news and the bad news may come hand in hand. A suspicious lump may turn out not to be cancer (good news) but instead is evidence of a glandular problem (bad news). A patient with a serious injury may make a full recovery (good news) but only after a grueling physical therapy regimen (bad news). Life can be messy; medicine even more so, and sometimes struggle and celebration can come in the same package.

When it comes to *your* health, longevity, and quality of life, I want to give you a little more. There is a famous Clint Eastwood Western called *The Good, the Bad and the Ugly*; I want to give you the good, the bad, and the extraordinary. So, after I give you the good and bad news, I'm going to give you the extraordinary news: a blueprint for reigniting your life like I did.

Let's start with the good news. Allow me to remind you of something that we forget all-too-often: Just by being alive right now, you have won the evolutionary lottery. You are a miracle. You are! I don't mean to sound so cliché, but it happens to be true. To be a human being alive today, you have inherited the genes and gifts of many generations of natural selection of those that come before you. You are also a survivor, a winner—you beat out more than three million sperm battling for life, but it was you who made it. This is no simple feat. Like every single human being on this Earth, you were born with greatness encoded into your genes.

Every human accomplishment is an example of what we are capable of. We have been gifted with the mental acuity to be able to put a man on the moon, the emotional intelligence to create great works of art, and a physical body capable of scaling the world's mountains. Every person who lives past one hundred is living proof that there is no artificial limit to how long we can live and even thrive.

All of us have abundant untapped potential for better overall health, greater human performance, and longer life. But the tensions of the modern world—from our morning commute, to our microwaved lunch, to our fifth cup of coffee—often keep us from operating at full potential. Perhaps most importantly, our society's definition of "success" does not match up with a healthy lifestyle.

So, here comes the bad news. The bad news is that there's a high probability that you may be suffering from a chronic disease right now, even if you haven't been diagnosed yet. Chronic disease comes in a wide range of dispiriting options—from diabetes, to high blood pressure, to arthritis, to cancer, to a multitude of autoimmune conditions. In fact, one of every two Americans has a chronic disease, and one in four has two (or more) of the eighty-plus chronic diseases officially recognized by the Centers for Disease Control and Prevention (CDC). These debilitating conditions have literally become national as well as global epidemics.

Conventional medicine is at advanced levels never seen before in history, and the United States currently spends more money on healthcare than we've ever spent and more money per capita than any industrialized nation. Yet we're also the unhealthiest we've ever been. Life expectancy in the United States has increased each year for the majority of the past 60 years, but the rate of increase has slowed over time, and life expectancy actually decreased after 2014 for a few years.[1]

Even the economic cost of chronic disease is staggering. According to the Milken Institute, the total cost of direct treatment for chronic health conditions totaled $1.1 trillion in 2016, or 5.8% of U.S. gross domestic product (GDP).[2] By adding in the indirect cost (i.e., lost workplace productivity), the total financial cost of chronic disease grew to $3.7 trillion, or 19.6% of GDP. That means that one out of every five dollars in the U.S. economy is spent on healthcare, with a large proportion of that going to the top three most costly conditions: diabetes, Alzheimer's disease, and osteoarthritis.

There's a famous story about the Dalai Lama. As the story goes, a reporter once asked the spiritual leader what surprised him most about humanity. He responded: "Man surprised me most about humanity. Because he sacrifices his health in order to make money. Then he sacrifices money to recuperate his health. And then he is so anxious about the future that he does not enjoy the present; the result being that he does not live in the present or the future; he lives as if he is never going to die, and then dies having never really lived."

If you're a high achiever, you probably know exactly what the Dalai Lama was talking about. You've worked hard and smart all your life, put in long hours to reach the top of your game, and perhaps you've even sacrificed a bit of happiness to get there. Now you find yourself stuck in neutral—lacking the energy, strength, and good health to continue along your life's journey. Your physical and mental health are suffering. Your relationships are suffering. Your inner spirit is suffering. YOU are suffering.

I know exactly what that feels like. I've been there. Let me tell you about how I shifted to a healthier state in my own life, how I took these lessons and combined them with my traditional and non-traditional medical

---

1   Steven H. Woolf and Heidi Schoomaker, "Life Expectancy and Mortality Rates in the United States, 1959-2017," *JAMA* 322, no. 20 (November 26, 2019): 1935-2032.

2   Hugh Waters and Marlton Graf, The Costs of Chronic Disease in the U.S. Executive Summary, (Santa Monica: The Milken Institute, 2018), Online PDF.

knowledge to develop my blueprint for better health, and how you can do the same.

My journey began when I made the decision to live a more authentic and purpose-driven life. And in this journey, I've discovered one of the most important lessons—health is a personal discovery process. As one begins to master their health, they discover their own personal power in all areas of their lives.

This is extraordinary news. Within you lies the answers to your own blueprint to achieve optimal wellness, peak performance, and longevity—to unlock your greatness to share with the world. I know this not only because I have seen it as a doctor but also because I have lived it. Within this book, I will show you how to embark on your own transformative personal health journey. If we change not only our health practices but also our definition of health, we are capable of a remarkable transformation—one that has ramifications that stretch far beyond our own lives. I envision a world where humans embrace a standard of health that enables us to be happier, live longer and more fully, and contribute our gifts to humanity with joy and intention. I believe that if we change our health, we will change the world. This is not hyperbole. I have seen how the practices I teach here for achieving optimal individual performance and health can be applied by teams, organizations, and businesses. That is incredibly exciting! I wrote the first edition of this book in the hope that my personal journey and my hard-won professional knowledge will help inspire others to realize that they are their own best medicine. That's still true and profoundly important. In this edition, I share what I've learned about how the same practices can benefit society.

Now that you've heard the good, bad, and extraordinary news, consider these questions: How would your life be different if you knew you could live an extra decade or two past what we currently think of as a healthy lifespan? What more would you do in your life, relationships, or business if you had more energy, physical vitality, and mental capacity as you age? What more would you be capable of? If the answers to these questions leave you feeling hopeful, energized, and motivated for the future, then you've picked up the right book.

To help you on your journey to Thrive State, I've put together some additional tools and assets you can use as a companion to this book in a free resource guide you can download at thrivestatebook.com/resources.

CHAPTER 1

HOW I REVERSED MY CHRONIC DISEASES

As a physician, I work with a lot of unhealthy people, and at one point in my life, I was an unhealthy person working with unhealthy people. I had type 2 diabetes and high blood pressure and, just like many of my patients, I took several medications daily. I had been practicing medicine for twelve years—and yet, I had the same problems that many of my patients did.

The worst part was that, in the back of my mind, I knew that I was responsible for the poor state of my health. Years earlier, I had made the choice—by what I ate and drank, what I did and didn't do with my body (e.g., sleep and exercise), and by how I managed my reactions to the things that I couldn't control (stress). It was not until a single experience with a terminally ill patient that I was able to break out of these old patterns and accept that I had the power to enjoy abundant health, wellbeing, and vitality.

My health discovery story actually begins with my journey as an infant fleeing with my family from postwar Vietnam. My Chinese grandparents fled from China to Vietnam during the height of WWII, and after the Vietnam war, our family was to flee again. When I was just a few months old, my parents scooped me up, along with a handful of our worldly possessions, and we boarded a boat with over two thousand other refugees sailing toward a better future. Our boat was anchored in Manila Bay for eight months... and it doesn't take a doctor to know that in a situation like that, disease and poor sanitation conditions can become life-threatening. People died. I nearly died myself, fighting a life-and-death battle with dysentery before I even knew how to speak. In fact, I was the only baby on the boat to survive. Later, we were transferred to a Philippine refugee camp, and after three months, a Catholic church sponsored our relocation to the United States—to Los Angeles, city of angels and second chances.

My family lived in Chinatown, a poor immigrant neighborhood in downtown Los Angeles. Having tested as "highly gifted," I was fortunate to attend a good school in a more affluent area of town. But being a poor Asian kid at a "rich-kid" school was no walk in the park. I was constantly teased and bullied for being different. For being poor. For the holes in my hand-me-down clothes. For the "stinky" food my mom sent me to school with. The other kids would say, "Go back home to your country, Chinky."

Those early experiences shaped me. I had revenge on my mind. Not the vindictive or violent type but rather the "I'll really show you when I'm famous" type of revenge. I vividly recall my revenge would be to become famous and inspire people like Tony Robbins, make people laugh like Robin Williams, and wow the audience like Mick Jagger. Then, I bumped into a bit of revenge reality. None of my heroes looked like me. There were no Asian motivational speakers, comedians, rockstars, or role models that I could pin my hopes on.

Coming home from school, I found myself wishing I were someone else. Someone who was taller... whiter... richer... lived in a different neighborhood... and had a more "American" family. I didn't know it at the time, but this childhood desire to be someone else—this feeling that I wasn't enough as myself—would dog me for years and would prove to be the seed of my adult illnesses.

Growing up in an immigrant household, my career ambitions of being a rockstar or a comedian were... discouraged. My mother gave me three career options: I could become an M.D., a D.R., or a physician. And for those of you who did not grow up with Chinese mothers, I should explain:

when I say that my mom gave me three options, I mean that those were my *only* three options!

So, I put aside my dreams of stardom and studied to be a doctor. Like the thousands of others who pursue an education in medicine, I worked day and night. In college, I studied biochemistry and cell biology, spending late nights in my dorm room or in the library cramming for the next test. I graduated from UC San Diego magna cum laude and was even the commencement speaker. But I had no time to rest on my laurels—my goals were still ahead of me. Next was the MCAT—the Medical College Admissions Test. More long nights, more studying... and more thoughts of the "revenge" I would obtain by being more successful than those who bullied me as a child.

Then it was medical school itself, and after that, a residency in internal medicine, followed by a residency in diagnostic radiology, followed by a fellowship in Interventional Radiology. I ground out long, hard hours, day after day, for years. And finally, after a full decade of education aimed at this one result, my work finally began to pay off. My career started to skyrocket. I was in a private group practice and became the Chief of Interventional Radiology at my hospital. My salary afforded me a fancy house and a fancy car, and I even flew around the world to give fancy medical speeches.

By many measures of life, I was now an unqualified "success." I had achieved my revenge—or so I kept telling myself. But I wasn't happy. And under my white coat, I was unhealthy and ashamed.

Not only was I overweight, but I had developed type 2 diabetes and hypertension and was taking several prescription medications, even drugs to help me fall asleep. I felt horrible, not just because I was sick but also because I was living a lie. I felt like such a hypocrite. Every day, I would ask myself, *How do I walk into a patient's room, look them in the eye, and tell them how to take care of their health, when I am not even taking care of my own? Who in their right mind is going to take (and more importantly, follow) medical advice from a walking, talking chronic disease statistic?* This was my internal dilemma—I was a success on paper, but I didn't feel like a success. They say that the best revenge is a life well-lived. Well, I had motivated myself with thoughts of this exact type of revenge—but even though I had money, prestige, and respect, I still did not have a well-lived life. In fact, some days it felt like the opposite. The harder I pushed myself, the sicker I got, and the more disappointed I felt.

This shame was compounded by painful developments in my personal life. I had put so much pressure on myself to perform at my job that I had neglected my relationships. I had been in a committed relationship with a woman who left me for someone else. I took this as a personal failure, one that I brought with me into the hospital. How could I be an authority on health for my patients when I didn't have my own life together?

And, of course, all of these embarrassments combined to demoralize and demotivate me. What was the point of working out or eating better? I didn't feel like anything was going to fundamentally change in my life or that I had a lot to look forward to. So why push so hard to be healthy?

One day, when I was feeling particularly sorry for myself, I prepared for my rounds. I went to meet one of my patients—Ishmael, a forty-three-year-old man with terminal pancreatic cancer who required ten liters of fluid be drained from his belly. I opened the door to his room, expecting to see a man in despair. After all, if I felt so terrible even when my life looked so great, then Ishmael must be really struggling with his situation. Or so I thought.

But Ishmael greeted me with a smile and an upbeat, "Hey, Doc! How ya doing, man?"

I couldn't understand the source of his positivity. This was a man who was facing the end of a life unjustly cut short—bed-ridden and in a state of constant pain. So, bewildered, I asked him, "Ishmael, why are you so happy right now?"

With a grin, he said, "It's easy, Doc. I'm so grateful to be alive. And every moment I'm here, I choose to spread love and joy."

Ishmael's words were so simple, but I felt as if I had just been shocked with a defibrillator. *Here's a man who's about to die, and he's reminding me how to consciously live. He's reminding me that no matter life's circumstances we find ourselves in, we always have a choice as to how we show up.*

In medicine, when a body's physiology is out of alignment, the heart can go into a dangerous or even fatal rhythm. But it's possible in many instances to shock the heart back into normal sinus rhythm, as if hitting the "reset" button. Similarly, my life was out of alignment, and Ishmael inspired me to press my reset button, which put me on the path to living the life I was meant to live—the life that included reversing my chronic diseases. Ishmael died soon after that conversation. But with just a few words, he changed my life. His attitude shocked me into a new rhythm.

Modern medical care is "symptoms-centric." We're so focused on managing symptoms with medications that we don't even think about eliminating the root causes of illness. Furthermore, many in the medical profession don't even give a second thought on *how* to get at the root cause. If there's a pill for a symptom, we prescribe it—whether it's for the sake of expediency or presumed patient satisfaction—because that's what we were taught in medical school. But these symptoms—elevated blood pressure, abnormal cholesterol levels, out-of-range blood sugars, insomnia, or pain—are most assuredly *not* telling us that more medications are needed. Instead, they're direct messages from our bodies begging us to take back our power and to step into the fullness of who we really are as amazing human beings.

And that's why I was sick. I was living a lie that denied who I truly was. Yes, I was this "successful" medical doctor, but I reached this place for all the wrong reasons. Even today, I'm embarrassed to admit what it took me years to acknowledge to myself: I didn't choose to be a doctor just because I wanted to heal people. Nor was it because my mother made me—though I will admit that it is a tough task trying to say "no" to my mother!

But no. I became a physician because I wanted to be respected. Even though, deep down, I didn't have enough respect for myself. I was still the young boy that the other kids used to call "Chinky" and taunt me for being poor, and who dreamed of being someone else. I used my white coat, with my name and the M.D. initials embroidered on it, to cover up for the "not enoughness" and shame I was feeling inside.

I had climbed a majestic mountain to success, only to discover that I had climbed the *wrong* mountain. Throughout life, I had followed the "recipe for success," only to realize that I was in the *wrong* kitchen. At home and at the hospital, I was expected to be serious, stoic, and strong, yet that wasn't the real me—at least, most of the time. I'm an artist and goofball who really enjoys making people laugh. To my detriment, I hid that part of me because, as one supervisor liked to remind me, "Dr. V... there's no humor in medicine."

After my encounter with Ishmael, I pressed the reset button—joyfully. I started small, with a couple changes to my daily routine that helped me lose a few pounds. Buoyed with the confidence of this early 'win,' I implemented changes in my diet, exercise, and sleep routine—changes which I will discuss throughout the book. But more than just changing my routine, I changed my attitude—I reignited and explored the good-humored artist within me, I reprioritized my time so that I was spending more of it with those I cared about, and I approached every interaction with gratitude and joy.

I pushed my personal boundaries: taking on more public speaking op-portunities—something I'd always enjoyed—and going further by working to create funny, inspirational web content for people I wanted to reach. I even hosted a series titled *Behind the White Coat*, a comedic talk show that blended health, education, and a touch of Hollywood. I felt like I had finally found an outlet for parts of my personality that I had suppressed for years. It was a truly gratifying and liberating experience. And, of course, it was the beginning of the journey that eventually reversed my chronic diseases.

In four to six months, I had lowered my blood pressure, reversed my hypertension, and cured my diabetes. I remember looking at the results of my blood work with stunned but joyful disbelief. It was a life-changing event. Better still, I was solely responsible for the turn-around. I had gone from feeling like an imposter to feeling a sense of genuine accomplish-ment—one that was free from any misplaced motives of "revenge" for the slights I had suffered in my past.

But that wasn't even the best part. The best part was that I now had proof of the concept that our everyday choices and our core purpose in life are our best medicine. I was a one-person testament to the power of joy and gratitude, and I could look my patients in the eye and say to them, in good faith, "I reversed my own chronic disease, so I know that you can too." Hypertension and diabetes are two of the most significant causes of mortality in American society today, and I had kicked them both. I had an important message to share with anyone willing to listen.

Austrian physician and Holocaust survivor Viktor Frankl said, "Between stimulus and response, there's a space. In that space is our power to choose our response. In our response lies our growth and freedom." This quote reiterates Ishmael's point for me. Our power, our growth, our freedom, and our health lie in the choices we make—moment by moment by moment.

By changing my attitude and my behaviors, I had reversed not one but two chronic diseases—hypertension and diabetes. Talk about physician, heal thyself! I had reached my ideal weight, and I had stopped taking the prescription medications, which, only months before, I had seen as essential to my health. I began to recognize that I had control over my own health—something that I had preached to my patients, but I hadn't truly believed until that point.

I knew I was on to something, and I knew I wanted to learn more. The real question for me—and I suspect, for you reading this book as well—isn't just how to reverse disease. It's how to perform at our best. It is how to have a longer, more meaningful, and (dare I say it?) *better* life. I resolved that my new state of health would represent the beginning, not the end, of my journey to a greater state of wellness. I began expanding my medical research interests, reading widely into areas of medicine that I had traditionally dismissed as not relevant to my practice. Nutrition, for example: despite the fact that so many patients go to their doctor for diet advice, the truth is that nutrition is all but ignored as a subject in medical school, despite its importance. I found myself approaching the field of medicine with fresh eyes, asking myself not only how I could treat sickness but how I could promote health.

Eventually, I pursued a Fellowship in Anti-Aging, Metabolic, and Functional Medicine with the American Board of Anti-Aging and Regenerative Medicine. I wanted to explore perhaps the greatest challenge in medicine, a question that stretches back all the way back to Pythagoras: how can we live longer?

It was through this fellowship that I began to develop my own expert understanding of the field of study that we call *epigenetics* ("*epi*" means above, and "*genetics*" refers to genes, or DNA), which explains how external factors—outside the genes themselves— actually control how our cells behave and, ultimately, our overall health and performance. Epigenetics shows us that our choices create the environment of our cells, also known as the *epigenome*, which in turn dictates how our genes are activated or expressed. Epigenetics is one of the newest and most exciting frontiers of medicine today, advancing our understanding of human health and longevity in ways that medical scientists previously thought impossible.

In the study of epigenetics, the first thing a doctor learns is how important environmental factors are to human health. More than 95 percent of the chronic diseases faced by Americans have lifestyle components. Getting adequate restorative sleep, eating nutritious foods, experiencing fulfilling personal relationships, and having a supportive community all contribute to whether or not we get disease. Our very thoughts and emotions contribute to both mental and physical health. This is something that the average person understands intuitively on some level... but only to a certain extent. We all know that our lifestyle has overall effects on our health, but we don't realize the extent to which it has tangible, demonstrable effects in our body. Epigenetics is a map to our body—an incomplete map that researchers and doctors are constantly drawing and redrawing—that illustrates the effects of our lifestyles.

As I studied epigenetics and other areas of integrative medicine, I was better able to understand my own personal health journey through the lens of medical science and ancient wisdom. Sure, I already knew the connection between, say, diabetes and sugary drinks, but I was learning how to more effectively diagnose how the non-stop red-alert work schedule of a large hospital inevitably damages the health of those who work there. I learned how important biomedical markers, like our hormone levels or our telomere lengths, are linked to elements that we dismiss as lifestyle factors: sleep, nutrition, exercise, and stress.

Furthermore, I began to better understand how living a purposeful life can have a beneficial effect on your health, an effect that manifests itself on a basic level. This all may sound simplistic or new-agey, but epigenetics research demonstrates that by tapping into the state of eudaemonic happiness—the joy you feel when you have deep meaning and purpose in your life—you activate the genes that give you better health, enhanced immunity, and decreased inflammation. On the cellular level, all biological, chemical, neurological interactions are in homeostasis (balance), and this creates optimal health and performance within each cell. When the body's cells are able to function optimally, we experience the same. By living life in congruence with your purpose—*why you are here*—you are gifted with abundant health, vitality, and optimal performance.

Even more significantly, when you are living in this eudaemonic state, your telomeres are better preserved. You may actually live longer because your cells are able to replicate more times without degrading. It's as if your body is rewarding you for living your truth and fulfilling your purpose.

But how do we know what our truth is? What our purpose is? The answer to that question is a far more complicated one, one that I wanted to explore for my own sake as well as for medical knowledge. I didn't want to just live a *longer* life. I wanted to live a *better* life.

This is why, in my quest to reach my own personal best for my health, I did not restrict myself to the halls of medicine. I also started studying self-optimization—attending conferences, reading books, and participating in seminars around the country with people who had dedicated their lives to examining these questions from psychological, sociological, and even spiritual perspectives. I started to access the ideas of people like Vishen Lakiani, Michael Bernard Beckwith, Lisa Nichols, Shawn Achor, Bruce Lipton, Joe Dispenza, and Tony Robbins; people who had deeply explored the psychology of happiness and wellness. I figured that these figures had already spent a *lot* of time examining the question of how to live a better life, and I'd be a fool to try and reinvent the wheel on my own!

Drawing from these self-optimization lessons, I explored my emotions, my mindset, and my relationships with others. I had long conversations with my parents, sharing honestly with them my childhood resentments and unanswered questions, hoping to deepen our relationships and reset broken dynamics. Growing up, my parents and I never hugged, and the words "I love you" were infrequent at best. Now, my father and I say "I love you" almost every conversation, and my mother cannot leave my house without "getting her hug in."

I worked on forgiving others that I felt had wronged me and seeking forgiveness for my own mistakes. I was building new habits and practices but ones that people associated more with spiritual meaning than physical health: meditation, daily affirmations, invocations of gratitude. But the results were that I felt better, more joyful, less stressed, and more energized. The health benefits spoke for themselves.

As I continued my explorations, I felt like I was straddling two worlds. In one, I was learning about telomeres, microbiomes, and mediator complexes. And in another, I was learning about forgiveness, intention, and living in the present. Yet it was obvious that each of these two worlds reinforced the other. True health is impossible without a sense of happiness and meaning, and in return, your happiness will make you healthier. These two different fields—functional/integrative medicine and self-optimization—were speaking different languages... but once I learned to translate, I realized that they were saying the same thing!

There is an ancient Indian parable about three blind men touching an elephant. Each man, feeling a different part of the elephant's body, thinks the elephant is something different. One man touches the trunk and thinks the elephant is a massive snake. Another feels the elephant's legs and thinks the elephant must be a tree. The third blind man feels the elephant's tusks and thinks that they are giant spears. The moral of the story is obvious: no one person or idea has a monopoly on the truth. We all have something to learn from each other.

I was one of those blind men. I examined the idea of human health from one framework—the framework of traditional Western medical training and practice. And through that framework, I have been able to understand so much about what makes us sick and what makes us well. But I haven't learned everything. With both integrative medicine and self-optimization, I have been able to enlarge my understanding. I'm still blind... I've just been able to examine several different parts of the elephant!

And as I learned, I found myself—almost unconsciously—developing a framework for synthesizing the knowledge I was gaining from so many different sources. I have always found that I learn better when I fit everything into one overarching idea; when I put the puzzle pieces into one cohesive whole. This new stage of my life was no exception. I began thinking of how to place the many different aspects of human health and wellness into a small group of major elements. Sleep, Nutrition, and Exercise would be a few of them, yes, but I would also include elements like Purpose and Community—issues that healthcare workers normally view as well outside of their area of expertise... but ones that can massively impact our health and longevity.

I began with over twenty BioEnergetic elements, but a framework where you have to remember twenty different pillars is not useful at all: I wanted something easy to remember because if you remember it, you are more likely to act on it. I eventually boiled these elements down to seven overarching areas: Sleep, Nutrition, Movement, Stress, Mindset, Relationships & Community, and Purpose. Once these foundational pillars fell into place, it was easy for me to recognize my strengths and my weaknesses—and not just my own, but my patients'.

I started applying the BioEnergetic Elements model to my concierge clients. It made for a useful and easy diagnostic tool—one that helped me identify my clients' issues far more quickly and accurately. Many patients come to me with health problems who are at their wit's end. They're getting eight hours of sleep, eating well, and hitting the gym or the exercise bike regularly. But they are also working twelve-hour days, barely seeing the sun, and using their free time to binge-watch Netflix. What does that mean for their stress? Their mindset? Their relationships with others? In other words, what does that mean for their health?

I have other patients who do everything right... almost. But they completely sacrifice one Element of their health. I've seen working parents who feel like they've gone years without a good night's sleep, or amateur sports fanatics who live to exercise but still eat like college students. Through the BioEnergetic Elements framework, it becomes easy to identify the problem: they are ignoring one major Element of their health and hoping that they can get away with it by excelling in other areas. But that's not how our bodies work.

This book is the result of my development of this framework—my examination of our seven pillars of health, our BioEnergetic Elements, alongside my guidance for how we can reach the Thrive State at both a cellular and a human level. But more than that, this book is a result of my journey—from achieving "success" by sacrificing my happiness and health to becoming a happier, healthier, and more authentic version of myself, who also happens to be a fitter, stronger, and smarter version as well.

Within the pages of this book, I will lay out my framework for a healthier and more fulfilling life—one in which your health and longevity is attached to greater purpose, community, and joy. You will learn more about my story, about the BioEnergetic Model, and about how to transition from the "Stress State" to the "Thrive State"—both on a biological level and on a human level. I will offer my synthesis of some of the most up-to-date research on the big questions: How do we live healthier? How do we live better? How do our environments and our life choices affect our health?

Throughout, I will be offering my thoughts on many of the contemporary discussions around health: everything from pesticides to Pilates, sleep cycles to psychedelics. There is a dizzying world of health-related information out there, and I want to help you parse through it all. But the point of this book is not to give you a comprehensive list of Dr. V-approved (or discouraged!) techniques and treatments. This book is not a recipe; it's a map. You do not have to follow any of my "instructions" to the letter. I just want you to use this book to help get you to where you're going.

To that end, I encourage you to read each chapter with an eye towards implementing one or two specific changes in your own life. Consider it the Dr. V Challenge. What can you immediately change in your own life in order to start practicing some of the ideas you will explore in this book? It's okay to start small. In fact, I highly encourage it! Make it easy! Baby steps are the key to implementing a new behavior, and it's the consistent stacking of these tiny habits that will create the momentum that will fuel your success.

I am not a health guru. I am just someone who has taken a substantial health journey of his own and who wants to share some of his insights as both a doctor and a former patient. As the result of my own journey, I'm experiencing the best physical and mental health and level of performance of my life thus far. My healing journey began with the simple choice to start accepting, loving, and living as the TRUE me. And right this moment, I tell you that the same is possible for you.

If you have symptoms, or you have a diagnosed disease, or you feel that your life is out of alignment, don't wait for a shock. If you could press the reset button right now, how do you envision the true you? How will you feel when you finally own the power of your choices?

I want to help you find out. Time to get your mojo back. Let's get to the Thrive State together.

CHAPTER 2

THE BIOENERGETIC MODEL &
7 BIOENERGETIC ELEMENTS

I developed my clinical practice as an interventional radiologist: a medical specialty using imaging technology to peer inside of the body and to diagnose and to treat disease with minimal invasiveness. I gravitated towards interventional radiology, as opposed to other types of radiology, so that I could spend time directly with patients, getting to connect with them personally as I planned their treatment strategies. Especially with the most difficult cases, people who are fighting for their lives, it can be hard to connect. But I'm a people person. I couldn't have it any other way.

Because of this, every once in a while, I feel myself getting a little stir-crazy when I'm staring at computer screens for long periods of time, trying to interpret my newest batch of tests. I have to remind myself that, as a radiologist, I get to use some of the most sophisticated technology available to modern medicine, all to answer perhaps the most basic question of human health: "What seems to be the problem?"

Even so, while these cutting-edge devices can detect and treat lesions, cancers, and other abnormalities, they don't give me the big picture—such as how vibrant or creative you are; how resilient or forgiving you are; whether you're holding onto emotional trauma; whether you live with joy, purpose, and passion in your life; whether you're contributing to the larger community or just taking from it.

At this point, I imagine you're asking yourself, *Why would a doctor need to know any of that personal stuff? What could it possibly tell Dr. V about me and my health?* Well, these factors make up your body's overall BioEnergetic State—or the energy/frequency/vibration that are broadcast to all of your cells with the instruction to either thrive or enter a disease state. This is the name of the game, dear reader: how to ensure that our body is in a positive BioEnergetic State and thus sending the right signals to our component cells.

At any given moment, you are a walking radio station, and the individual component cells of your body are the audience for that radio station. You're not only broadcasting out to the world—you are broadcasting inward, to your own cells, and even to your own genes. And in fact, they're not just listening—they are taking their marching orders from the signals they receive moment by moment.

So, what determines the content of your "broadcast"? Everything. Every input into your body is energy. This includes the food you eat, the sleep you accrue each night, and the exercise you eke out for yourself during the day. But it also includes your mental state, your environmental stressors, and even the tangled everyday emotional experiences you have. These signals will drive your genetic expression on how to behave and dictate the direction of your cellular activity. As a result, you have incredible power over whether you call upon your cellular and genetic self to either flourish (the Thrive State) or hunker down as if besieged (the "Stress State" or "Survive State").

Every input is energy that comes into our body, and our body's functions are merely a series of biochemical processes. You give the body an input, and it will eventually translate the energy from that input into concrete molecular and biochemical changes. Think of your hormones, your growth factors, your chemical mediators and enzymes. These are all signals that induce your cells to act in a certain way. We are, all of us, just the collective output of that chemical conversation.

The BioEnergetic model begins by identifying all of these inputs. From a patient-oriented perspective, the BioEnergetic model allows us to diagnose how to improve a patient's health at a basic level—focusing not on the symptomatic results of their health problems but on the core reason(s) for their ill-health. Each of my BioEnergetic Elements, then, can be seen as an input, a major constituent element of the "signal" that we are sending to our own cellular microenvironment and to our own genes. Seen through this prism, it becomes far more obvious that seemingly abstract concepts like happiness or community can have concrete and tangible effects on our physical health—particularly, if we feel that these ideals are absent from our lives.

Since I was, in fact, once a patient myself, I'd like to think that I have a little insight into the patient experience—being told that pharmaceutical drugs were the prescribed treatment for the hypertension and diabetes I had developed. These were the same treatments I had learned in medical school to be the "standard of practice" or "standard of care." Surely, when it came to my own health, I didn't want drugs to be "standard." And so, it wasn't until I started applying the principles of this BioEnergetic Model that I was able to reverse all my chronic diseases and be in the best state of health and performance in my life. Most chronic diseases, including cancer, develop slowly from a disordered relationship between cells and their cellular community—a result of poor signals from their environment, or what I describe as being in a low BioEnergetic—"stress" or "survive"—state. As I mentioned previously, one in every two Americans has a chronic disease, and one in four has at least two chronic diseases. This national and global epidemic must be addressed if humans want to continue their existence with any degree of success.

Signs Your Health May Be in Trouble

- Excess belly fat ("spare tire")
- Elevated blood sugar levels
- Digestive problems (gas, bloating, constipation, diarrhea)
- Excessive tiredness or exhaustion
- Emotional problems (depression, anxiety)
- "Brain fog"
- Food or airborne allergies
- Skin problems (psoriasis, eczema)
- Gum disease
- Erectile dysfunction in men

Some people just don't feel well, even if they've never been formally diagnosed with a named chronic disease. They sort of know that something isn't right but often chalk it up to a hectic work schedule, a demanding boss, or just being in a job they really don't like. They may say to themselves: *If I change jobs, I'll feel better* or *If I get a raise, I won't feel so stressed.* Unfortunately, these are just excuses—excuses that are deleterious to one's physical and mental health. Stress, or rather the **reaction** to stressful situations, over time, can be a significant factor in the development of chronic disease. When individuals are chronically ill, they simply cannot function at their highest potential. Thus, my aim with this book is to help you, the reader, no matter where you are on the spectrum of "not feeling well." Whether it's been years or decades, you can recover.

Let's backtrack slightly and examine the American workforce. For most people, our work years are the time of life that we consider most productive. Yet this "productivity" seems all-too-often to come at the cost of our own health. And, even worse, our workaholic culture arguably makes us *less* productive, given the effects of chronic disease on our ability to be sustainably productive. Employees with cardiovascular disease, type 2 diabetes, and hypertension, as well as depression and other mental health issues, are negatively impacting workforce productivity and increasing healthcare costs. Meanwhile, the direct medical costs associated with chronic disease will exceed $1 trillion annually, or 80 percent of the total healthcare spending in the U.S.[3] As I'm sure you can recognize, these statistics represent a tangible diminishment of the quality of life for so many Americans... including, perhaps, you!

But chronic disease is not the only boogeyman out there. There is also the prospect of physical and mental decline. So, let's talk about it. Here is a question for you: when was the last time you thought about SCD? Wait just a moment... what the heck is SCD? Perhaps, if I called it "pre-Alzheimer's," more of you would have perked up. SCD, or subjective cognitive decline, is a type of mental impairment characterized by more frequent episodes or worsening memory loss and/or confusion that affects an individual's ability to care for him/herself. Generally, we think of memory impairment disorders affecting mostly older adults, but recent research suggests that younger adults—those in their productive years—are also affected. While one in nine adults aged forty-five and older (11.2%) self-report memory problems, one in ten adults aged forty-five to fifty-four (10.4%) report SCD. What's even more alarming is that one in six and a half adults (15.2%) who also have a chronic disease report SCD.[4]

Nowadays, nothing seems to scare people more than the possibility that they may develop Alzheimer's disease, and those sobering statistics should be a call to action. You may be underperforming at work, need to lose fifteen pounds, lack meaningful relationships, or feel depressed a little more than usual, and still not feel that kick in the pants that motivates you to change—your very own Ishmael moment. But when it comes to one's memory, that's a redline for many people. Maybe it is a redline for you. After all, Descartes taught us that "I think, therefore I am." If this is

---

3   "What Is Chronic Illness?" PBS, www.ppbs.org.

4   Christopher A. Taylor, Erin D. Bouldin, and Lisa C. McGuire, "Subjective Cognitive Decline Among Adults Aged ≥ 45 Years — United States, 2015 – 2016," *Morbidity and Mortality Weekly Report* 67, no.27 (2018): 753-757.

true, then cognitive decline is so threatening to us because it signals a loss of self—of self-control, self-identity, and self-awareness.

Whatever the reason for not functioning at your highest potential, I want you to know that my vision for better health and full-potential functioning can be yours too. I want everyone to not just *live at life* with a day-to-day existence but to *thrive at life*, every moment of every day. When you're thriving at life, you'll have better memory and brain function, more consistent energy levels, more meaningful personal relationships, more satisfying sexual relationships, and better physical health and vitality.

BioEnergetic Medicine

BioEnergetic Medicine is the study of the flow and transformation of energy in living organisms. The BioEnergetic Model for Health synthesizes knowledge gained from observing high-performing entrepreneurs and athletes, new science from epigenetics, integrative and functional medicine, and biohacking, as well as anti-aging and regenerative medicine. The underlying premise of this model is that life is energy, we are all energetic beings, and everything in the universe is made up of energy, which interacts with other forms of energy. Human beings are made up of cells, and each cell is made up of energy—both physical and non-physical energy. Cells work together, utilizing energy to form tissues. Then, tissues function together through energy to form organs. Organs communicate with other organs through the energy of hormones, peptide (protein) molecules, and the nervous system to form the body. And our outer bodies have different receptors to take in various energies—light, sound, food, and emotions such as love and anger—and transmute them back into each of our cells. If you look at the big picture, our cells are constantly being directed by various energies emanating from and within their cellular environments.

Now you're probably wondering about DNA—the double-helix you first learned about in high school science class. *Isn't DNA, or my genes, what instructs my cells?* The answer is *technically, yes* but also *no*.

The science of epigenetics tells us that the fate of each cell is not fully determined by the genes that reside in it but rather how these genes interact with the energy (signals) from their cellular environment—what I have termed the **BioEnergetic State**. The physical form of the BioEnergetic State is called the **epigenome**, which is the multitude of biochemical compounds that instruct the genome. The environmental inputs determine which genes are turned on or off and how a cell will behave from moment to moment. Given the right BioEnergetic cues, a cell will flourish and grow, be rich with energy, live longer, and support the growth and healing of cells around it. Given the wrong cues, the cell will be inflamed, diseased, and potentially destructive to neighboring cells. The good news is that we are ultimately in control of our cellular environment through our lifestyle choices, including our thoughts—whether positive or negative.

To illustrate the concept of epigenetics, let's take a set of hypothetical male twins (twins always make for good studies in the research world). Here's the scenario: Identical twin boys were born to a young couple whose financial situation only allowed them to adequately care for one child (Twin #1), and so one of the twins (Twin #2) was put up for and adopted within days of his birth. The twins are genetically the same; their cells contain the same genes they inherited from their biological parents. Although they will grow up separately with different lifestyles, they will have the exact same eye color, hair color, and other physical features They will also have genetic predispositions, such as heart disease (from Dad, whose male family members all died before age fifty of heart attacks) and obesity (from Mom, whose three siblings have type 2 diabetes); there is no evidence of mental illness on either side of the family. Both twins have loving parents and stable home environments, but only Twin #1 was breastfed; Twin #2 was formula-fed.

According to the genetics model, both twins will develop heart disease and obesity like their biological parents and be on the path to type 2 diabetes and early death. Genetics is the nature component of the equation while epigenetics is more of the nurture component. Epigenetics could be the overriding factor in why one or both of the twins do not develop the chronic diseases that they're predisposed to get. For example, Twin #2's parents are aware and concerned about their son's genetic inheritance, so they go all out to protect their son by raising him a healthy environment; they eat nutritiously, enroll Twin #2 in after-school sports, minimize his screen time, participate in family-fun activities, and educate him about sexually transmitted infections. Even though Twin #2 could not reap the benefits of breastfeeding, his parents made every effort to feed him high-quality organic foods as an infant and as a youngster. Twin #2 grows up, maintains a healthy lifestyle, has a rewarding career, and a successful marriage; at age forty, he has no clinical evidence of heart disease or diabetes despite being five pounds over his ideal body weight.

Twin #1's parents are much more resigned that their son will suffer the same health destiny as themselves. They don't make any concerted effort to maintain a healthy lifestyle, although Mom believes breastfeeding is the best gift she can give to her son and does so for a full year exclusively. Twin #1 is a healthy baby and rarely gets sick, but he's pudgy throughout most of his childhood, has borderline-high fasting blood glucose levels by high school, and really starts packing on the pounds during college. Twin #1 likes junk food, spends a lot of his free time playing video games alone, hates his job, and has been unsuccessful at dating; at age forty, he is fifty pounds overweight and has been diagnosed with prediabetes and arterial plaque.

The twins' genome determines their physical features and is a singular entity because they both have the same DNA blueprint. It is their individual BioEnergetic State, or epigenomes, that are vastly different. The BioEnergetic State allows for their individual experiences to affect the expression of their genes. It's as if you gave two identical sets of interior floor plans to two different architects—one from the East Coast (Twin #1) and the other from the West Coast (Twin #2)—and you asked them to create the elevation plans (e.g., roof line, exterior finishes, etc.), based on their individual experiences of growing up on opposite ends of the country, their finished plans are quite different. Twin #1 fashions a steep-pitched roof; double-pane, hurricane-strength windows to accommodate Vermont's heavy winter snowfall and occasional high-wind event; and a brick exterior for strength (and no earthquakes). Twin #2 fashions a slight-pitched roof for rain drainage (but no snow); double-pane, tinted windows (for sun protection); and a stucco-covered exterior to better survive a California earthquake. The interior layout of the two houses is exactly the same, but the exteriors are very different.

Epigenetics is more than simply nature versus nurture, but it does show us that how we live life can overcome the genetic hand we're dealt. Whether it's with behavioral changes (e.g., diet, exercise, sleep), which elicit positive physical well-being, or with positive mental consciousness (e.g., stress management, mindset), which elicits emotional well-being, we can prevent the "bad" genes from being expressed. As we learn more about epigenetics, we will be able to minimize certain chronic diseases and achieve our fullest potentials as human beings.

DR. V – RECOMMENDED READING

To learn more about epigenetics, I recommend *Super Genes* (2015) by Deepak Chopra, MD and Rudolph E. Tanzi, PhD This highly praised book "illustrates the interplay of nature and nurture using cutting-edge science and [they] argue persuasively that adapting one's lifestyle can maximize the potential to transcend the inherited susceptibilities handed down to us from our parents." (James Guesella, PhD, Director, Center for Human Genetic Research, Massachusetts General Hospital) Drs. Chopra and Tanzi teach readers how to utilize their minds to instruct their genes to heal their bodies.

Dr. Joe Dispenza, DC teaches that the body is the subconscious mind and our subconscious thoughts transmit signals to the cells about their environment.[5] For example: you feel anxious about an upcoming presentation

---

5   "The Official Website of Dr. Joe Dispenza," drjoedispenza.com.

at work and you get "butterflies." The stress signals from the subconscious cause your blood pressure to go up, and the butterflies are now causing unpleasant gut symptoms. Suddenly, you experience the urge to use the bathroom. This is a temporary situation, and once your presentation is over, your blood pressure returns to normal and the butterflies go away. But if you're constantly sending "worry" or "doubt" signals, then your cells respond with initiation and/or perpetuation of disease.

Of the numerous environmental signals that can potentially affect the behavior of a cell, I have identified seven primary BioEnergetic Elements that contribute most to the BioEnergetic State (frequency or vibration) of the entire body. I call them the 7 BEEs. They are Sleep, Nutrition, Movement, Stress and Emotional Control, Mindset, Relationships/Community, and Purpose.

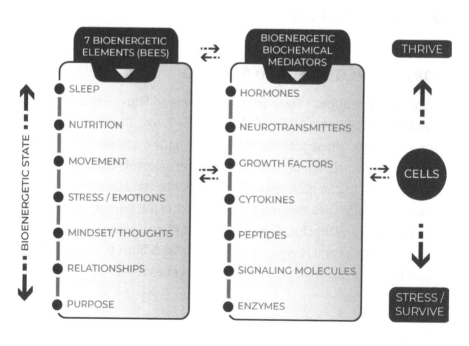

Thrive State & Chronic Health

Wouldn't it be amazing if we could say, "I'm chronically healthy," or "I've got chronic health." Well, it's certainly possible and probably easier than you might imagine. In the optimal BioEnergetic State—what I call the *Thrive State*—your cells receive instructions to grow, heal, and... thrive. Your sex and well-being hormones increase, giving you a sense of joy, happiness, and heightened libido. You experience improved immunity, making you better equipped to fight off pathogens and toxins. Your cells' power plants, the mitochondria, have improved efficiency and energy output; mitochondria produce ATP (adenosine triphosphate), which supplies energy to drive the processes within living cells and maintain human life. When your cells have more energy, you also have more energy. You'll enjoy the health benefits of lower levels of (bad) inflammation and longer telomeres, the DNA endcaps that protect your cells from aging. The *Thrive State* puts your body in a realm of regenerative growth and healing, which translates to vitality, optimal performance, and longevity.

Stress State and Chronic Disease

Conversely, in a depressed or suboptimal BioEnergetic State, the opposite happens. I call this the Stress or Survive State. In the Stress or Survive State, our cells are state of defense, and energy is diverted from biological mechanisms for growth and healing to mechanisms for protection. Inflammation is the key biological process in the Stress State. Cells age quicker and are unable to repair and regenerate themselves. The mitochondria are less efficient at generating ATP, so the body has less energy to operate optimally. Lower levels of sex and "feel-good" hormones (e.g., serotonin) and higher levels of stress hormones (e.g., cortisol) lead to mental imbalance and unhealthy physical symptoms. Inflammation increases and becomes chronic, leading to autoimmune disorders and other chronic diseases. Telomeres shorten, leading to degradation of your DNA. The *Stress* or *Survival State* puts the body into overdrive and exhaustion, which not only prevents optimal functioning but hastens the development of disability, pain, and premature death.

The body's physiological response to the stresses from daily life can mimic that of our ancient ancestors running away from a saber tooth tiger; your nervous system diverts from parasympathetic to sympathetic. Your blood thickens and clots easier, and inflammation increases to protect you from a potential flesh injury. Your immune system shuts down—because why try to protect yourself from viruses and cancer if you're potentially breakfast for a predator? Blood diverts from your visceral organs to your skeletal muscles so you can run away from this predator, but this impairs the function of organs like your gut and kidney. While this Stress/Survive State is a useful physiological response for occasions that really threaten life—i.e., running away from a predator or a response to bleeding from a car/motorcycle accident—its chronic activation in today's world of perceived threats (mean bosses, spoiled milk, overworking, deadlines) creates the backdrop for the rise in our nation's chronic disease statistics.

An optimal BioEnergetic State—the Thrive State—is always the goal, so let's examine how you can transition from the *Stress State* to the *Thrive State*. The seven BioEnergetic Elements—Sleep, Nutrition, Movement, Stress and Emotional Mastery, Mindset, Relationships/Community, and Purpose—create the BioEnergetic State and epigenome for our cells and energetically influence each other. As you begin to improve one Element, you'll see it's easier to elevate the frequency/vibration of the other six Elements. For example: when your sleep improves, in terms of both quality and quantity, it rebalances your hormones (growth and sex hormones) and other physiological processes, which will give you more energy to exercise, which, in turn, can lower your stress levels. Lower stress levels allow you to better digest and extract nutrients from the foods you eat. This, in turn, will further yield optimized neurotransmitters and hormones, which can elevate your emotional states. This gives you fuel to work on your purpose and contribute to your community. It's a positive feedback loop. Your elevated BioEnergetic State will also raise the states of the people around you.

It's a "virtuous cycle." The same thing also happens at the cellular level; healthy cells elevate the states of their less-healthy counterparts.

The BioEnergetic Model for Health		
	THRIVE STATE	STRESS/ SURVIVE STATE
Mitochondria/ cellular energy	More efficient	Less efficient
Telomeres/aging	Longer/cells live longer	Shorter/more cell aging
Inflammation	Decreased	Increased
Organ Function	Optimized	Diminished
Hormones	Higher levels of sex and feel-good hormones, lower levels of stress hormones	Lower levels of sex and feel-good hormones, higher chronic elevations of stress hormones
Nervous System	Parasympathetic dominant	Chronically elevated sympathetic states
Microbiome	Optimized	Propensity for dysbiosis and "leaky gut"
Cellular immunity	Increased	Decreased
Chronic disease	Prevent/reverse diseases like Alzheimer's, dementia, and other chronic conditions	More prone to diabetes, hypertension, autoimmune disorders, cancer
What "mind" are we operating from?	Heart-centered, conscious mind (Soul/Spirit/Purpose centered)	Head-centered, subconscious programs (EGO centered)

Now, it's easy to see how Sleep, Nutrition, Movement, Alleviating Stress and Emotional Control, and Mindset—the physical, emotional, and mental components of the energetic elements—can benefit the individual. These five Elements are integral to every health education or wellness program ever created and have undoubtedly been drilled into you by your doctor, workplace wellness coordinator, or life coach. Get more restful, restorative sleep. Eat more fruits and vegetables. Do some physical activity every day. Control your stress. Think positive. But despite your best efforts, you may have felt as if there was something missing.

One can never achieve his or her highest BioEnergetic potential unless Community and Purpose—the spiritual component of the energetic elements—are included, and there is a reason why our genes are wired this way. This mutual, symbiotic dependence was the only way multicellular life evolved. We are who we are today because cells worked together in synergy to form the complexity of life on Earth. Our cells—and we ourselves —are meant to thrive as individuals, of course, but ultimately as a group so that we can give back and elevate the community for the collective good.

For example: a heart cell *has* to be the very best heart cell in order to fulfill its purpose and pump effectively as possible to deliver oxygen and nutrient-rich blood throughout the body. The brain, liver, and lungs receive this life-sustaining nourishment granted to them by the cells of their other fully functioning co-organs. If a heart cell decides, *I'm not going to follow my purpose. I want to filter blood like a kidney cell, not pump blood*, not only will this cause circulatory collapse, but the cellular process of transforming one type of cell into another is what leads to cancer. The whole organism will thrive only if every cell fulfills and contributes its unique purpose to its fullest potential. And that can only happen when a cell receives signals from a high BioEnergetic State.

Integrating Purpose & Community into Your Life

Picasso once said, "The meaning of life is to find your gift. The purpose of life is to give it away." Now, ask yourself what your gift is. If nothing comes to mind immediately, begin by thinking about the things that bring you joy—gardening, singing in the choir, playing basketball with friends, cooking for extended family, or playing chess in the park. Your gift or gifts are the activities and people in your life that you love and that spark joy and passion—whether you're actively involved or just thinking about them. This gift comes naturally to you— it's encoded in your DNA—and it usually feels effortless when you engage with it. When you serve your Community doing that thing(s), well... that's your Purpose. Put simply, your purpose is really to share your authenticity and joy with others.

For example, one of my favorite activities in the world is something that a lot of other people dread: karaoke. If you live in Los Angeles and you tend to go to karaoke bars, there's a good chance you will see me there, belting my heart out. And don't worry, I only pick some of the best karaoke songs. We're talking Lionel Ritchie, Kenny Rogers, Frank Sinatra... and, of course, the Righteous Brothers. I sing a pretty decent "You've Got That Loving Feeling," if I do say so myself.

Now, this doesn't mean that I should be a professional karaoke singer. I'm not that good, as my friends occasionally remind me. But karaoke is an activity that is best done in groups; it is an activity that revolves around entertainment and spectacle, and it is an activity where a little corniness and enthusiasm is not just acceptable, it's downright encouraged. And those are the things I love about karaoke. Once I came to recognize that these elements are the building blocks of my joy and passion—the building blocks of my gift—I had a better lead on my Purpose.

When you add Purpose and Community into the mix, you begin experiencing a higher BioEnergetic State and your thrive potential expands. Not only do you wake up rested and refreshed, but you actually wake up excited and you make good choices throughout the day. When you feel good about yourself, it's much easier to make healthy choices—whether it's skipping the sugar-laden donut, or taking the stairs instead of the elevator, or meditating on your lunchbreak instead of smoking a cigarette.

The BioEnergetic Model of Health informs us that our state of health and performance is largely controlled by energetic inputs we give our cells by the choices we make. Going from a low to optimal BioEnergetic State usually means choosing to cultivate positive emotions such as trust, love, and gratitude instead of indulging in fear, anger, or guilt. In doing so, we choose to act from our hearts instead of our heads, and choose to serve WE instead of me. After all, we are simply cells in a larger body of humanity, and whether we realize it or not, we have a choice as to how we live, how we feel, and how we impact the lives of others. We can choose to be the cancer cell that abandons community and is destructive to humanity, or we can choose to be the healthy cell that thrives and gives back to the collective body to move humanity forward. In Chapter 11 I share exciting examples of how I have seen the BioEnergetic State elevate not just individuals, but organizations.

ACTIVITY: Rev Up Your BioEnergetic State

Close your eyes. Imagine and feel an energy field surrounding your body as a vibrating, pulsating white light. Take in a deep breath and as you exhale slowly... think of one thing in your life you'd like to change in order to elevate your BioEnergetic State. Maybe it's getting more sleep, eating more vegetables, taking a walk every morning, or seeking out more joy. Take in another deep breath and as you exhale... envision yourself performing that activity. Now feel your energy field radiate and expand. It's pulsating with more intensity. It knows that just doing that one thing alone makes it easier to shift the energy of other Elements. Take in another deep breath and as you exhale, expand your white light so that the energy fills the room and the positive vibrations reach anyone and everyone around you. Take in another deep breath and as you exhale, expand the light even further... so that your energy envelops your neighborhood, town, or city. And now the entire planet. Feel yourself connected to the planet. Now open your eyes and feel the energy of your immediate space. When we collectively raise the energy within ourselves, as a group, or as a community, we'll not only heal ourselves, but we can heal the world.

5 to Thrive

1. The BioEnergetic Model of Health provides a framework to understand the relationship between disease (the Stress/Survive State) and abundant health, longevity, and optimal performance (the Thrive State).

2. The genes you inherit may predispose you to health or disease, but how your genes are expressed (turned on/off) is controlled by your Bioenergetic State (epigenome), which is largely determined by your choices/habits.

3. Although there is an infinite amount of energetic inputs that can potentially affect cellular behavior, there are 7 primary bioenergetic elements (BEEs) that contribute most to the BioEnergetic State: Sleep, Nutrition, Movement/Exercise, Stress and Emotional Mastery, Mindset, Relationships/Community, and Purpose.

4. The BEEs are energetically connected, and improvement in one BioEnergetic Element lends to improvement in all of the others, which synergistically elevates the BioEnergetic State (energetic resonance).

5. Use this book as a blueprint and write down a few ideas that you can implement with each chapter. Start small and implement the idea that requires the least amount of effort. Consistent implementation will turn this idea into a habit. Then implement the next small idea; this will build energetic momentum, which will stack, and before you know it, you become the product of all the habits that will put you into the Thrive State.

CHAPTER 3

SLEEPING FOR SUCCESS

When it comes to sleep, I'm probably just like you and the millions of people who at one point or another in life underestimated the *value* of a good night's sleep. I spent years sacrificing my sleep in pursuit of my goals: late-night study sessions, day-long work shifts at the hospital, and (I'll admit) the occasional way-too-late social night thrown in. I figured I could sleep when I was dead... or at least when I wasn't so busy. But even with all my medical training, I didn't really appreciate how insufficient sleep can't simply be solved at a later date. The chronic effects of lack of sleep are more significant than we acknowledge, as is the *health value* of high-quality, restorative sleep. And so, there's a reason that SLEEP is the first BioEnergetic Element I'll be discussing. If you get no further than to the end of this chapter, you will at least be ahead of the game and on the path to your Thrive State.

Again, I ask, do you want the good news or the bad news about sleep first? The bad news is probably what you'd expect—a lot of people are sleep deprived. A 2018 study in the Centers for Disease Control and Prevention's (CDC) *Morbidity and Mortality Weekly Report* estimated that nearly

35 percent of American adults don't get the recommended seven or more hours of sleep per day on a regular basis.[6]

Although there are differing opinions on exactly how many hours are necessary—and even some evidence that too much sleep can also be bad for you—the American Academy of Sleep Medicine and the Sleep Research Society recommend at least seven hours nightly for adults who are between 18 and 60 years old for optimal health. Anything less is associated with an elevated risk of developing a chronic health condition. And, by the way, only the actual time spent sleeping counts; you could be in bed for eight hours and spend two of those fully awake, tossing and turning.

Short-term sleep problems, such as daytime sleepiness and inability to fully concentrate, can lead to accidents and silly mistakes. And let's face it; you're probably a bit of a grouch if you don't get enough sleep. We've all had the occasional bad sleep situation and generally recover with a daytime nap or some weekend catch-up sleep. Health professionals agree that occasionally not getting a good night's sleep isn't going to make you sick, but chronic sleep deprivation has been linked to hypertension, obesity, type 2 diabetes, heart disease, and stroke as well as anxiety and depression. So, by all accounts, poor sleep is a public health crisis.

But, there's good news. We have learned so much about the physiological aspects of sleep that we know how to fix the problem of sleep deprivation and can offer solid recommendations to improve one's sleep and, ultimately, one's BioEnergetic State. Understanding is key to solving any problem. But unlike with diet or exercise, the average person does not really think about *how* to sleep better—what routines and habits they can pursue to ensure they get not only more sleep, but higher quality sleep. So, let's examine the phenomenon of sleep, starting with how your body responds when you sleep.

---

6   "1 In 3 Adults Don't Get Enough Sleep," CDC Newsroom, Centers for Disease Control and Prevention, last reviewed February 16, 2016.

The Circadian Rhythm & Sleep

In the simplest terms, you can think of circadian rhythm as your 24-hour internal clock, or your sleep/wake cycle. It cycles between states of sleepiness and alertness, and for most people, there are two distinguishable periods of a low or lower energy state—one around 2:00 a.m. to 4:00 a.m. and another around 1:00 p.m. to 3:00 p.m. These correspond to the times when (1) most people, aside from "night owls" and "morning larks" are asleep, and (2) post-lunchtime, when the idea of taking a nap (the traditional siesta) feels pretty good. When you're all caught up on sleep, these low-energy states are less noticeable (i.e., you're not craving a post-lunch nap); but if you're sleep-deprived, you'll experience a bigger swing between feeling alert and feeling sleepy.

Circadian rhythm is controlled by the hypothalamus, which is influenced by cycles of lightness and darkness. When it's dark outside (nighttime), the eyes signal the hypothalamus that it's time to feel tired. The brain signals the pineal gland and other tissues to start secreting melatonin, and the adrenals to stop secreting cortisol, which induces the sensation of being

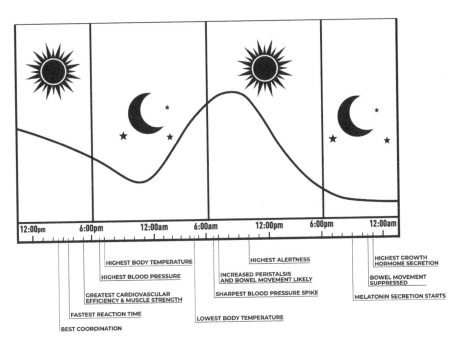

41

tired. In other words, your brain is making you feel tired so that your body can enter its regenerative state as you sleep. The following morning, when the sunlight enters through your bedroom window or the alarm clock goes off, the eyes signal the hypothalamus that it's time to stop feeling tired. The brain signals the body to stop secreting melatonin and begin secreting cortisol, which induces the sensation of wakefulness. A few yawns, a good stretch, and you're ready to start your day. That may seem like an overly simplistic explanation, but I think it gives a basis for understanding where things can go wrong if there are insults to your normal circadian rhythm.

There are plenty of factors that can disrupt your circadian rhythm, including those that you can control (e.g., going to bed and waking up at the same time every day) and those that you may have less control over (e.g., daylight saving time, jet lag). Optimizing your circadian rhythm involves regular sleep habits and good sleep hygiene, which I'll define and discuss later. Keep in mind that if you binge-watch your favorite Netflix series until 2:00 a.m., you're likely to feel sleepy and have a bit of brain fog the next day—neither of which are good for your BioEnergetic State.

Normal Sleep Cycle

Throughout the night, the brain cycles through five distinct sleep stages, with each cycle lasting between 90 and 120 minutes. These cycles consist of REM (rapid eye movement) sleep and non-REM sleep. REM sleep is characterized by rapid, shallow, and irregular breathing; temporary paralysis of the arm and leg muscles; and rapid eye movement (eyes darting back and forth). During REM sleep, brain waves are quick and less synchronous, and this is when you dream; the first REM sleep period occurs about 70 – 90 minutes after you first fall asleep. Non-REM sleep and deep non-REM sleep (delta stage) are characterized by slow, synchronized brain waves and no eye movement. Humans spend about 80 percent of their sleep time in non-REM.

Stage 1: Light Sleep – the period between wakefulness and sleep; muscles begin to relax, and the eyes move slowly. You can drift in and out of sleep and/or be easily awakened.

Stage 2: Sleep – the onset of non-REM sleep; breathing and heart rate slow and become more regular; eye movement stops; body temperature drops; and cortisol levels dip slightly. Brain waves become slower and process less complicated tasks.

Stage 3: Deep Sleep – non-REM restorative sleep period when slow delta brain waves first appear; muscles are relaxed, and blood pressure drops. Hormones (e.g., growth hormones) are released. The body repairs bone and skin tissue.

Stage 4: Delta Wave Deep Sleep – non-REM restorative sleep period consisting primarily of delta waves; blood flow to the muscles increases. Increased blood flow plus growth hormones are necessary for muscle tissue repair and growth and for restoration of physical energy (to be used the next day).

Stage 5: REM Sleep – brief period of REM sleep; heart rate and body temperature increase. The brain is very active, and dreams can be intense or vivid.

Unless you suffer from obstructive sleep apnea or another sleep disturbance, four or five complete sleep cycles will allow your body to repair itself, and you'll wake up feeling refreshed the next morning. The goal is to ensure complete cycles and not be awakened in between stages. For example: if you awaken in Stage 4, you're likely to be groggy and disoriented. Plan your sleep cycles and set your alarm clock accordingly.

Poor Sleep & Hunger-Regulating Hormones

Let's examine the hunger-regulating hormones—ghrelin and leptin—which are influenced by insufficient sleep and can play a role in the development of obesity, insulin resistance, and type 2 diabetes. Ghrelin is often referred to as the "hunger hormone," as its primary function is to increase appetite; it's manufactured in the gut and secreted when the stomach is on "E" (empty). Ghrelin travels through the bloodstream to the hypothalamus, which then tells you to feel hungry so that you'll seek out and eat food... and eat more and more and more. All those excess calories get stored as fat.

Conversely, leptin is the "satiety hormone," which reduces appetite; it's manufactured by adipose (fat) cells and in the small intestine. Leptin also acts on the hypothalamus by which it sends the "F" (full) signal so that you'll stop eating. Problems arise when the two hormones are out of whack—high ghrelin levels and low leptin levels. Sleep restriction has this very effect, and a persistent state of hormonal imbalance can initiate a vicious cycle of overeating, which leads to weight gain and insulin resistance.[7]

The graphic on the following page illustrates the potential mechanism by which obesity can be the end result of chronic sleep loss (i.e., insufficient or poor-quality sleep). Sleep loss causes daytime tiredness, which results in reduced physical activity and a lower basal metabolic rate, so the body burns fewer calories. More hours spent awake provide more opportunity to eat calorie-dense foods, so the body stores more calories as fat. Hormonal changes not only increase appetite but also influence food choices—typically processed and high-calorie snack foods.

Sleep & Chronic Disease

Sleep, or lack thereof, exerts a significant impact on the development of certain chronic diseases, many of which are linked to premature death. Certainly, no one wants to die prematurely, and so there has been a lot of interest surrounding the goal of improving sleep as a means to prevent diseases that rob us of our Thrive State. Insufficient sleep also impacts patients' abilities to manage the chronic disease(s) they've developed, whether or not sleep issues actually caused the problem. In other words, not sleeping well

---

7   Bo Xi et al., "Short sleep duration predicts risk of metabolic syndrome: a systematic review and meta-analysis," *Sleep Medicine Reviews* 18, no. 4 (August 2014): 293-7.

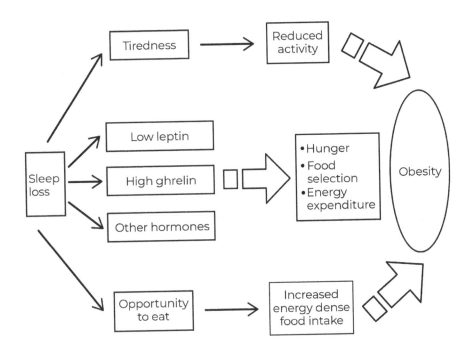

can impede the day-to-day management of some diseases. Furthermore, many of the chronic diseases discussed on the next page go hand-in-hand with each other, and it is not uncommon to see patients who are obese and have type 2 diabetes, cardiovascular disease, and mental health challenges simultaneously.

Another consideration in the development of chronic disease is that of epigenetics and how sleep affects "clock genes."[8] Clock genes do more than determine whether someone is a morning lark or a night owl; they impact cognitive function, immunity, inflammation, and metabolic health. A lack of sleep doesn't just disrupt the natural circadian rhythm but affects the expression of these clock genes via DNA methylation (the "turning on" or "turning off" of specific genes). The goal then, is to strive for adequate, quality sleep as part of the overall BioEnergetic plan to attain the Thrive State.

8   Irfan A. Qureshi and Mark F. Mehler, "Epigenetics of Sleep and Chronobiology," *Current Neurology and Neuroscience Reports* 14, no.3 (March 2014): 432.

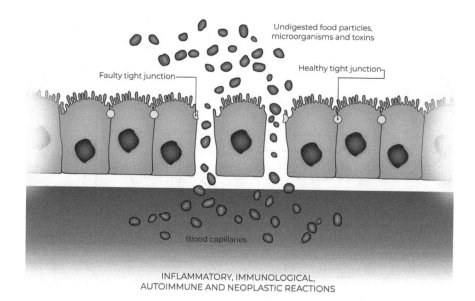

INFLAMMATORY, IMMUNOLOGICAL,
AUTOIMMUNE AND NEOPLASTIC REACTIONS

Obesity

Numerous epidemiologic studies have detailed an inverse association between sleep duration and excess body weight in various socioeconomic populations and in all age groups. A 2019 meta-analysis showed that shorter sleep duration significantly increased obesity risk. For each one-hour decrease in sleep lower than seven hours, the obesity risk increased 9%.[9] It's quite possible that sleep-compromised, obese adults, in fact, got on the path to obesity during their youth. Because childhood and adolescence are key times for brain development, insufficient sleep can impact the hypothalamus' regulation of appetite and energy expenditure.[10] If young people don't "outgrow" their weight issues, they're poised not only to enter adulthood obese but to develop additional chronic diseases, including cardiovascular disease and type 2 diabetes if they haven't already.

---

9   Qionggui Zhou, Ming Zhang, and Dongshang Hu, "Dose-response association between sleep duration and obesity risk: a systematic review and meta-analysis of prospective cohort studies," *Sleeping and Breathing* 23, no.4 (December 2019): 1035-1045.

10   Shahrad Taheri, "The link between short sleep duration and obesity: we should recommend more sleep to prevent obesity," *Archives of Disease in Childhood* 91, no.11 (November 2006): 881-4.

I remember one patient of mine—let's call her "Sarah." Sarah was forty-five, overweight, and struggling with the fact that she just couldn't seem to lose the weight. During my original consultation with her, she laid out all the ways that she had tried to shed those stubborn pounds. She was eating moderate portions, exercising, and cutting out the junk foods. But it didn't seem to have any effect. She was clearly distraught—she was doing everything "right" but wasn't getting the right result.

Like I said at the beginning of the book, however, you can be strong at all but one of the BioEnergetic elements and still suffer adverse health effects. Each Element is a load-bearing pillar: it can't be removed without the entire building crashing down. For Sarah, the Element that she was ignoring was sleep. Once I drilled down on Sarah's sleeping patterns, it became obvious to me that her lack of sleep was likely connected to her inability to lose the weight that was bothering her so much. On a practical level, no new diet or exercise regimen was going to solve the problem. Sarah needed her z's. So, I gave her my doctor's orders: a new sleeping schedule, eight hours, every night. And, lo and behold, with sleep came the weight loss she had been working so hard to achieve!

So many of us work so hard to lose weight—we sign up for grueling exercise classes or punishing diets. But one essential element to weight loss is something that isn't a punishment at all—a restful night's sleep.

Insulin Resistance

Insulin resistance—when your body cannot utilize the insulin produced by the β-cells in the pancreas—is the catalyst for increasing blood glucose levels. Over time and without lifestyle intervention, insulin resistance can precipitate the development of type 2 diabetes and cardiovascular disease. Sleep hours—too few or too many—are associated with insulin resistance and are believed to be a substantial link in the metabolic development of type 2 diabetes.[11] Sleep-deprivation studies in healthy, non-diabetic indi-

---

11   D van Dijk et al., "Associations between sleep duration and sleep debt with insulin sensitivity and insulin secretion in the EGIR-RISC Study," *Diabetes & Metabolism* 45, no.4 (November 2018): 375-381.

viduals have reported decreased insulin sensitivity and decreased β-cell function; one study showed insulin resistance could be induced with just a single night of partial sleep deprivation.[12]

Type 2 Diabetes

Researchers have found a link between insufficient sleep and an increased risk of developing type 2 diabetes.[13] Both sleep duration and sleep quality were strong predictors of *Hemoglobin A1c* (HbA1c), the standard by which glycemic control is measured. Research suggests improving sleep could be a potential management tool for patients with type 2 diabetes to help improve day-to-day glucose control and HbA1c levels. Similar results were found in patients who had type 1 diabetes.[14]

Cardiovascular Disease

Cardiovascular disease—atherosclerosis, hypertension, and heart failure caused by obstructive sleep apnea—have been linked to the body's inflammatory response to poor sleep. The exact cellular mechanisms have been difficult to pinpoint, but a 2019 study identified an interesting new piece of the puzzle. There is a brain hormone that regulates the production of inflammatory cells in bone marrow, which helps protect against blood vessel damage due to inflammation. Poor sleep quality or frequently disrupted sleep—as with sleep apnea—inhibits this anti-inflammatory mechanism.[15]

A lack of adequate, good-quality sleep is also an indirect causal factor in cardiovascular disease. When poor sleep interferes with the hunger

---

12   Esther Donga et al., "A single night of partial sleep deprivation induces insulin resistance in multiple metabolic pathways in healthy subjects," *The Journal of Clinical Endocrinology & Metabolism* 95, no. 6 (June 2010): 2963-8.

13   Kristen L. Knutson et al., "Role of Sleep Duration and Quality in the Risk and Severity of Type 2 Diabetes Mellitus," *Archives of Internal Medicine* 166, no.16 (September 2006): 1768-1764.

14   Sirimon Reutrakul et al., "Sleep characteristics in type 1 diabetes and associations with glycemic control: systematic review and meta-analysis," *Sleep Medicine* 23 (July 2016): 26-45.

15   Sarah Crunkhorn, "Sleep protects against atherosclerosis," *Nature Reviews Drug Discovery* 18 (March 2019): 254.

and satiety hormones ghrelin and leptin, the propensity to overeat leads to weight gain, which often leads to obesity and type 2 diabetes. (This connection between sleep, weight gain, and cardiovascular disease may help explain why, when I put my patient Sarah on her sleep regimen, her weight loss coincided with a lowering of her high blood pressure). The risk of atherosclerosis and hypertension is particularly dangerous if the excess calories are supplied by high-sugar, processed, and fast foods.

Depression

There appears to be a bidirectional relationship between sleep quality and depression or depressive symptoms, although it's difficult to say for certain whether this relationship is causal, and the research can be difficult to interpret.[16] Experiencing sleepless nights over an extended period of time may contribute to anxiety or depressive symptoms. Long-term insomnia can also be a sign of clinical depression. Additionally, individuals who have existing chronic disease(s) are prone to depression due to the heavy toll these conditions can take on one's physical, mental, and financial health. Continually being in the Stress State may induce sleep problems—either too little or too much.

Sleep Helps Propel Us into the Thrive State

Sleep is critical to repair and rejuvenation of the body's cells and tissues. We often underestimate sleep's value until chronic sleeplessness reminds us—usually in a not-so-good way. Sleep is a restorative process during which tissues repair themselves; cells synthesize proteins; growth hormones are secreted; and the brain removes its metabolic waste, consolidates memories, and processes new information. Success of these physical and cognitive processes is essential to the Thrive State, and high-quality sleep of appropriate duration is imperative.

---

16   João Dinis and Miguel Bragança, "Quality of Sleep and Depression in College Students: A Systematic Review," *Sleep Science* 11, no.4 (July – August 2018): 290-301.

Sleep Hygiene

Similar to the general concept of hygiene (bathing, shaving, hand washing, etc.), sleep hygiene encompasses habits or regular behaviors that improve the quality of nighttime sleep as well as promote daytime alertness. The Goldilocks rule of sleep hygiene is to get the right amount of sleep, not too little and not too much. Although sleep needs vary with age, health status, and lifestyle factors, the National Sleep Foundation has issued general recommendations. See the chart below.

Sleep Recommendations for Healthy Individuals	
Newborns (0 – 3 months)	14 – 17 hours
Infants (4 – 11 months)	12 – 15 hours
Toddlers (1 – 2 years)	11 – 14 hours
Preschoolers (3 – 5 years)	10 – 13 hours
School-aged children (6 – 13 years)	9 – 11 hours
Teenagers (14 – 17 years)	8 – 10 hours
Young adults (18 – 25 years)	7 – 9 hours
Adults (26 – 64 years)	7 – 9 hours
Older adults (65+ years)	7 – 8 hours

General Rules of Sleep Hygiene

1. Regular physical activity. (MOVEMENT – one of the 7 BEEs)
2. Avoiding stimulants or disruptive foods too close to bedtime. (NUTRITION – another of the 7 BEEs)
3. Getting adequate exposure to natural light during the day.
4. Taking a nap occasionally but limiting it to no more than 30 minutes, unless you get a full sleep cycle in.
5. Adhering to a regular, relaxing bedtime routine.
6. Immersing yourself in a pleasant sleep environment.

7. Going to bed and waking up at the same time every day.

8. Avoiding blue light before going to bed.

Now, I'll discuss each component of sleep hygiene in greater detail. Firstly, take note of how the BEEs all mutually reinforce one another—good nutrition and regular physical activity contribute to better sleep, which in turn provides a strong foundation for the other BEEs. None of these elements are siloed from each other.

Secondly, take note of the *sleep enhancers* and *sleep disruptors* and determine which ones you can modify so that you'll get a better night's sleep. Start by keeping a sleep diary that includes time you wake up, go to bed, how well you slept, and how you feel during the day. As you begin to improve your sleep quality and duration, you notice a difference in your energy levels, daytime productivity, and overall sense of well-being. It's all part of the transition from the Stress State to the Thrive State. And from my own personal experience, it feels REALLY good.

Regular Physical Activity / Exercise – Get Moving!

You don't need to run a marathon to get a good night's sleep. As little as ten to twenty minutes of moderate aerobic exercise—walking, jogging, swimming, or cycling—can improve nighttime sleep quality. For the best sleep, do some type of physical activity every day, and if you have health limitations, break your exercise into smaller sessions throughout the day. A side benefit to regular exercise is that it can promote weight loss and decrease the risk of obstructive sleep apnea.

We're not sure why exercise exerts a sleep benefit, but several theories have been proposed. First, exercise increases body temperature, and the corresponding post-exercise drop in temperature may promote falling asleep. To take advantage of this benefit, afternoon or early evening moderate aerobic exercise is

Dr. V's SLEEP Rx: Add exercise time and duration to your sleep diary. After a week, check for any patterns that indicate your ideal time to exercise.

recommended. Strenuous exercise close to bedtime isn't a good idea for most people, but since everyone is different, feel free to experiment with the timing of your workouts. Second, depending on the time of day exercise is performed, it may cause a shift in the circadian rhythm that favors nighttime sleep. If you experience frequent insomnia, this strategy may help. Lastly, any type of regular physical activity can improve sleep by decreasing anxiety, mental stress, heightened arousal, and depressive symptoms.

Sleep enhancer or sleep disruptor? Regular physical activity and structured exercise are sleep enhancers.

Nutrition – Ban the Stimulants & Sleep-Disrupting Foods!

Probably the worst thing you could do to ensure a bad night's sleep is to artificially stimulate your body too close to bedtime. You may want to go to sleep because you have to go to work in the morning, but your body's not having it. Foremost, smoking is a no-no. Nicotine is a neurotoxin and is bad for your brain and body in every way possible. Caffeine, on the other hand, is somewhat of a grey area, so no personal judgments here. I certainly enjoy my morning joe as much as anyone else. So, knowing that caffeinated beverages can affect sleep quality and duration, it's critical that you set a "caffeine curfew" so your body can metabolize and rid the body of caffeine before you hit the sack. For most people this is usually around two o'clock in the afternoon. If you're particularly sensitive to caffeine's effects, you may need to have your last latte before noon.

Certain foods and beverages can be disruptive to sleep because they trigger indigestion and heartburn. These include rich or heavy foods, fatty or fried foods, spicy foods, citrus fruits, and carbonated beverages. If this happens to you, avoid consuming them too close to bedtime and eat smaller portions. Ideally, avoid eating any large meal two to three hours before going to bed and don't eat anything except a light snack one hour before bed.

Dr. V's NUTRITION Rx: Include any negative food experiences in your sleep diary. That way you'll know whether it's a one-off or if you should avoid certain foods.

As for alcohol, a nightcap or few drinks can make you sleepy initially, but the effects are typically short-lived. You wake up feeling out of sorts, unable to get back to sleep, and sleep poorly when you do manage to fall asleep. The best advice is to curtail your drinking at least three hours before you intend to go to bed; this "alcohol curfew" allows time for your body to metabolize the alcohol and minimize the impact on sleep. Also, drink plenty of plain water to help the body flush out the alcohol metabolites (waste) quicker.

Two dietary supplements—magnesium and glycine—may actually help improve sleep. Magnesium is an essential mineral that has a wide range of functions in the human body. It helps maintain healthy levels of gamma-Aminobutyric acid (GABA), a sleep-promoting neurotransmitter. Magnesium-rich foods include dark leafy greens, sunflower and sesame seeds, cashews, almonds, broccoli, squash, legumes, dairy products, meat, unprocessed whole grains, chocolate, and coffee. Glycine is an amino acid that exerts a calming effect on the brain in preparation for sleep. It also helps lower nighttime body temperature so you can sleep better. The best dietary sources of glycine include meat, fish, eggs, milk, cheese, and legumes.

Sleep enhancer or sleep disruptor? Nicotine, caffeine, alcohol, carbonated beverages, and heavy, fatty, spicy, or acidic foods are sleep disruptors. Magnesium and glycine are sleep enhancers.

Expose Yourself... to Natural Light

Sunlight exposure during the day (and darkness at night) helps keep the circadian rhythm on track so your body knows when it should be sleeping and when it should be awake. The optimal time for your optical receptors and skin to catch some outdoor rays is between 6:00 a.m. and 8:30 a.m., for about 15 to 30 minutes. If you're not an early bird or it's the dead of winter and you're far north of the equator, sun exposure at later times of the day is fine. But, if you can't get outside at all, stand near a window and allow the sunlight to shine on your exposed skin.

Dr. V's SUNLIGHT Rx: Exercise for 20 to 30 minutes in the sunlight between the hours of 6:00 a.m. and 8:30 a.m. for maximum benefit.

Sleep enhancer or sleep disruptor? Exposure to sunlight, even if filtered through a window, is a sleep enhancer.

The Purr-fect Catnap

If you feel tired during the day, a 20- to 30-minute nap can help improve mental alertness, concentration, and performance. Take a cue from your feline (or canine) friend and doze off intentionally; that's infinitely better than unintentionally dozing off while you're driving. Napping won't make up for consistently poor sleep, but the occasional nap can help tide you over until the following night. Don't rely on napping to get you through the day and limit naps to no more than 30 minutes, unless you can get in a full sleep cycle; otherwise, you can wake up groggy.

Sleep enhancer or sleep disruptor? The occasional short nap is a sleep enhancer, but frequent napping can be a sleep disruptor and may signal a serious health problem.

Dr. V's NAPPING Rx: Record naps in your sleep diary; look for any patterns of excessive napping and consult your doctor.

Relax. Sleep. Repeat.

Following a regular relaxing routine at bedtime helps you de-stress after a long day and tells the body that it's time to get ready for sleep. It could be as simple as washing your face, brushing your teeth, and putting on pajamas, but for others, their bedtime routine may entail a few more rituals—taking a warm (not hot) bath or shower, meditating, stretching, listening to relaxing music, journaling, reading a book, or having sex and achieving orgasm.

Sleep enhancer or sleep disruptor? A relaxing bedtime routine is a sleep enhancer, but one that is non-relaxing and creates anxiety or wakefulness is a sleep disruptor.

Dr. V's RELAXING Rx: Find the bedtime routine that works best for you and don't assume screen time is relaxing (more on that topic to follow).

Sleep Environment Determines Sleep Quality – Choose Wisely.

If you've spent time successfully relaxing before bedtime, but your bedroom is full of "noise" and the mattress is lumpy, you probably won't get a good night's sleep. Maximum sleep quality depends on a pleasant sleep environment. Room temperature should be a cool 60 to 68 degrees, ideally without the constant loud humming of fans or jarring noise as AC units start up. The mattress and pillows should be of appropriate firmness and fabric (dogs are not considered pillows). Sheets, bedding, and pajamas should keep your body warm or slightly cool, but not cause you to overheat and wake up sweating.

Light from external sources—lamps, nightlights, the power button on the cable T.V. box, your neighbor's house, or even the moon—can make it difficult to sleep. Turn off which lights you can and block the rest with blackout curtains or eye shades. If you still use a digital alarm clock, cover it with a towel; if you use your phone as your alarm clock, turn it face down. Also, disable its noise-generating features—turn off alerts, turn down the ringer, or, better yet, turn it off completely if you can.

And now for the controversy... PETS. If you're having problems getting quality sleep or feeling well rested, I would recommend keeping the dogs, cats, rabbits, iguanas, and all God's other creatures out of the bedroom. They may provide some emotional comfort, but their presence is generally more of a hindrance to good sleep. If you feel that your pets must be in your bedroom, they should sleep in their own beds, not yours. A 2017 study evaluating sleep efficiency with one dog in the bedroom found that it was better if the dog was elsewhere in the room, rather than under the sheets.[17] Certainly, if you wake up every time your dog(s) rolls over, your sleep is interrupted; likewise, he'd probably prefer his own bed because he wakes up when you roll over. Additionally, pets can also introduce allergens,

---

17   Salma I. Patel et al., "The Effect of Dogs on Human Sleep in the Home Sleep Environment," *Mayo Clinic Proceedings* 92, no. 9 (September 2017): 1368-1372.

insects, and feces into your bedding which can trigger allergies or make you sick.

Furthermore, under the category of "all God's other creatures" falls the spouse or bedmate who snores like a freight train. Unless both parties are heavy sleepers, this noise can hinder the non-snorer's sleep, so it may be advisable for one party to relocate to another room for the comfort and benefit of both parties. If obstructive sleep apnea is suspected, a professional evaluation is warranted.

Dr. V's SLEEP ENVIRONMENT Rx: Treat your sleep environment the way the global environment should be treated—clean and pristine—for better quality sleep.

Sleep enhancer or sleep disruptor? Distractions, including light, sound, temperature, and pets are sleep disruptors. Your sleep environment is what you make it, so with some modifications, you can turn these disruptors into enhancers.

Set a Sleep Schedule & Stick to It.

Be a creature of habit by going to bed and waking up at the same time every day. The circadian rhythm relies on and works better with consistency. Even if your bedtime varies, try to ensure that your wake time is consistent, as this helps the body know when you should be awake (daytime) and asleep (nighttime). The benefits of observing a fixed wake time include:[18]

- Easier to wake up in the morning
- Less morning sleep inertia (the irresistible desire to go back to sleep)
- Easier to fall asleep at night
- Decreased sleep deprivation
- Fewer naps
- Reduced caffeine dependence
- Improved alertness
- Sharper focus and short-term memory

---

18 Brandon Peters, "First Step to Better Sleep: Wake Up at the Same Time Every Day," Verywell Health, May 13, 2020, verywellhealth.com.

- Brighter mood
- Less irritability
- Decreased pain
- Better immune system function
- Better safety and job performance
- Safe and attentive driving

Dr. V's SLEEP SCHEDULE Rx: You might be tempted to cheat a little on the weekend, but making the effort to stick to the same wake hour on the weekend as during the week will pay off in the long run.

Sleep enhancer or sleep disruptor? Following a consistent sleep schedule is definitely a sleep enhancer.

Do a Screen Dump Before Bedtime.

I saved the best for last because it's so ubiquitous in today's world and perhaps the most difficult habit to change. Screens are—computers, smartphones, iPads, televisions, even the Wi-Fi-enabled refrigerator that lets you know when you're out of milk. These devices emit artificial blue light that stimulates your body to increase secretion of daytime hormones (e.g., cortisol) and decrease secretion of nighttime hormones (e.g., melatonin). It's like they're telling you that you should be awake, when, in fact, you should be preparing for sleep (or actually in bed asleep). When your circadian rhythm gets out of whack, you have difficulties falling asleep, staying asleep, and you wake up tired from sleep deprivation. Turning off ALL screens a full 90 minutes prior to bedtime will help normalize cortisol and melatonin levels, thereby permitting a good night's sleep.

* Some research suggests that blue light may be dangerous for eye health by damaging the photoreceptors.[19] It has been suggested that the amount of blue light received during one's lifespan could be a contributing factor to the development of age-related macular degeneration (AMD). Thus, use of "blue blockers," glasses which block blue light, could offer some protection against AMD. I have my own pair of blue blocker glasses which I use at home!

And yes, I'll be honest—I had difficulty doing this in my own life. I am as addicted to my phone as anyone else. But since I went screen-free in the evenings—actually, I don't check my phone after 9:00 p.m.—I haven't

---

19 Gianluca Tosini, Ian Ferguson, and Kazuo Tsubota, "Effects of blue light on the circadian system and eye physiology," *Molecular Vision* 24, no. 22 (January 2016): 61-72.

been tempted to go back. After all, that email you check right before going to sleep… are you really going to answer it right then, or are you going to wait until the next morning anyway? Be kind to yourself and give yourself a little space from the distractions of the world.

Sleep enhancer or sleep disruptor? Blue light from our favorite technology devices is definitely a sleep disruptor.

Dr. V's SLEEP Rx:
If you absolutely must use your iPad at nighttime, get a blue light blocker or wear blue light blocking glasses.*

Now that we've covered the first BioEnergetic Element, how do you rate yourself? How do you rate your sleep? Do you get close to the recommended number of sleep hours? Are you currently more affected by sleep disruptors or sleep enhancers? Where can you improve? Are you ready to commit to better sleep? Getting to the Thrive State doesn't happen overnight, but it does begin with a good night's sleep.

Finally, I want to end each of these next several chapters with a challenge: take something from this chapter and try implementing it into your routine tonight. For SLEEP, perhaps it's getting thirty minutes more of natural light in the beginning of each day, or putting the phone away by a certain time each day, or—horrors!—kicking Fido out of the bedroom.

You can commit to *encouraging* a positive routine or habit or to *discouraging* a negative one. I think of it as falling into two camps: BioEnergetic Enhancers, which strengthen our BioEnergetic Elements, and BioEnergetic Detractors, which weaken (or at least potentially weaken) them. For sleep, BioEnergetic Enhancers include regular exercise, good nutrition, natural light, and stress management. BioEnergetic Detractors include drugs of all types, even down to the humble cup of coffee, and stress.

As you look at these Enhancers or Detractors, you may find yourself coming up with your one change to implement tonight. It doesn't have to be big. It just has to be a change that you seriously commit to.

5 to Thrive

1. Optimal sleep contributes to the Thrive State, which, in turn, gives you abundant health, longevity, and the optimal mental/physical/emotional performance you desire.

2. Lack of sleep is associated with poor performance and a host of chronic conditions, such as obesity, depression, cardiovascular disease, and some cancers.

3. General rules of sleep hygiene are: regular physical activity, avoiding stimulants or disruptive foods, getting natural daylight first thing in the morning, smart napping, regular bedtime routine, regular sleep schedule, and avoiding blue light before bed.

4. If you're having a hard time getting a good night's sleep, keeping a sleep diary will help you determine what factors are influencing your sleep, either positively or negatively.

5. Safe natural supplements that promote relaxation and sleep are magnesium and glycine.

For additional resources on how to optimize sleep, including sleep trackers, blue light blocking glasses, and other biohacks, visit thrivestatebook.com/resources.

CHAPTER 4

WHAT THE F*#% SHOULD I EAT?

Most of us can probably agree that the topic of nutrition can be quite all-encompassing, if not overwhelming. Just about *everybody* who's anybody or wants to be somebody in the field has written a nutrition—or dare I say "diet" book—touting the latest theory on weight loss and propelling them to instant fame. The books that we rushed out to buy, only to find that now they're sitting on a bookshelf collecting dust or somewhere on your Kindle, never to resurface. This chapter is about the second BioEnergetic Element—NUTRITION—with less emphasis on "diet" and more emphasis on the principles and benefits of healthy eating. Fueling your body and brain for maximum functioning potential is on par with sleep and is critical to achieving your Thrive State.

So, once again, I'll begin by asking, "Do you want the good news or the bad news about nutrition first?" The bad news is probably what you already know but would rather not accept—a lot of people are fat, or to put it nicely, over-fed. This may include you or someone you love. Some years ago, I included myself in that category—a Stress State—but worked to overcome it and achieved my Thrive State.

Along with being overfed, a majority are under-nourished, meaning that their daily nutrition is not supplying high-quality micronutrients their brain and bodies need for optimal functioning. It's akin to a vehicle that requires premium fuel; you can fill it with regular-grade gasoline, and it will get you from place A to place B, but its engine may not last as long as it would if you used premium-grade gasoline. Someone who is overfed simply stores the excess calories (energy) from food as adipose, or fat tissue. But don't think that if you're thin, you're off the hook. Your body may not be getting the nutrition it needs to reach the Thrive State. Furthermore, poor eating habits over a lifetime can lead to a malnourished body and, in some instances, cause disease.

Resetting Eating Habits

During my own journey from Stress State to Thrive State, the biggest change I made in my life had to do with what I ate. Days after my fateful meeting with patient Ishmael, when I realized I wanted to make a serious change in my own life, I asked myself where I should start. And the answer boiled down to one word: sugar.

By that point, I was actually going out of my way to put more sugar into my body. I was starting each day with five or six pumps of pre-sweetened creamer in my coffee. I'd follow that up with another couple of caffeine-meets-sugar cups of coffee throughout the day, and then switch to energy drinks towards the end of my shift. I told myself that it was just to push past the lack of sleep, to simply make it through another high-stress day. But habits—both good and bad—are developed by doing the same thing, over and over again, for a long time.

Meanwhile, the other healthcare workers and I were eating whatever snack food we could lay our hands on. Junk food is convenient. It's pre-packaged, easy to eat quickly, and it usually gives you that instant sugar rush that your body mistakenly believes it needs. Which is why it was perfect for a medical resident working in a high-energy, long-hours, non-stop major hospital. And by perfect, I mean that it was convenient, not that it was in any way good for us.

So, it was no surprise when—only a few months before meeting Ishma-el—I was diagnosed as diabetic. I had already started taking blood pressure medication to control my hypertension. I remember feeling this moment of exhaustion, when I realized that my newest diagnosis meant another pill that I would have to take. That extra pill began to represent the extra burden of my diabetes: the stress added to my already-stressful life.

This is one of the two reasons I chose to have my first step towards my Thrive State be cutting out sugar. I had the carrot of a healthier and hap-pier life hanging before me, but I also had the stick: I was a diabetic, and I needed to reset my relationship with sugar fast.

But that wasn't the only reason I started with cutting out sugar. I knew that if I wanted to make a change in my life, I needed to start with a single, simple habit. Just as I had created my daily habit of drinking two-to-three cups of pre-sweetened coffee, I could break that habit: slowly, by making a choice every day to forego the sweetener.

The master of habit formation is author James Clear, and his book *Atomic Habits* is a must-read for anyone looking to take greater control over their own habits. One of the most profound take-aways from Clear's work is how much our personalities are informed by our daily habits.

You are, on some level, the amalgam of the thousands of habits you re-enact every day. What time you set your morning alarm for. The route you take to work. How you take your lunch break. The weekly shows you watch. When you normally go to sleep. All of these choices shape our lives, even though none of them ever *feel* that momentous.

Like Aristotle once wrote: "We are what we repeatedly do. Excellence, then, is not an act, but a habit."

I knew that I could refrain from pumping that sweetener into my coffee, if I just put my mind to it. That was the first task I set for myself, the first habit to break. I had created the habit myself, and I could unmake it myself. And as I progressed—a week without creamers or energy drinks, then two weeks, then three—I felt a growing sense of confidence that I really could reset my body. This confidence helped buoy me, and it became easier to establish new habits—with food, especially. From cutting out sugary drinks,

I moved on to cutting out processed food from my diet. From there, it was making commitments to eat more organic vegetables and to make healthy choices for my protein sources. Eventually, I had transformed my diet.

That entire transformation started with a single first step. So, as you read through the following sections, give a thought to your own daily habits: what you can change, and where you could start? It doesn't have to be anything big, and, in fact, I encourage you to start small...as long as you promise yourself that you won't stop at just one change!

The Difference Between Overweight & Obese

Medical and health practitioners utilize the Centers for Disease Control and Prevention's (CDC) definitions to classify patients as overweight or obese.[20] People fall into either category when their body weight is higher than what is considered a healthy weight for their particular height. Body Mass Index (BMI) is the screening tool to assess body fatness; although BMI does not measure body fat directly nor does it diagnose obesity, the higher the BMI, the more fat a person is considered. BMI corresponds well with other more accurate and invasive tests to measure body fat directly and is also a good predictor of poor health outcomes, including death.[21,22] BMI is calculated by taking a person's weight (in kilograms) and dividing it by his or her height (in meters) squared.

$$BMI = weight\ (kg)\ /\ height\ (m)^2$$

20   "Defining Adult Overweight and Obesity," Overweight & Obesity, Centers for Disease Control and Prevention, Last reviewed June 30, 2020, www.cdc.gov.

21   Qi Sun et al., "Comparison of dual-energy x-ray absorptiometric and anthropometric measures of adiposity in relation to adiposity-related biologic factors," *American Journal of Epidemiology* 72, no. 12 (December 2010): 1442-54.

22   Katherine M. Flegal and Barry I. Graubard, "Estimates of excess deaths associated with body mass index and other anthropometric variables," *The American Journal of Clinical Nutrition* 89, no.4 (April 2009): 1213-9.

According to the CDC:

- BMI less than 18.5 = underweight
- BMI is between 18.5 and 25.0 = normal weight
- BMI is between 25.0 and 30.0 = overweight
- BMI is 30.0 or greater = obese

Obesity can be further subdivided into:

- Class 1: BMI of 30.0 to 35.0
- Class 2: BMI of 35.0 to 40.0
- Class 3: BMI of 40 or greater. Class 3 obesity is considered "extreme," or "severe," or "morbid" obesity.

In recent decades, there has been a significant increase in the number of Americans who are obese, who are younger when diagnosed with obesity, and who are living more of their lives with obesity. Statistics vary greatly as to the quantitative impact of obesity on life expectancy (i.e., number of years lost). In a 2014 study sponsored by the National Institutes of Health, researchers reviewed 20 published studies and determined that class III obesity (BMI of 40.0 – 59.0) was associated with an increase in the number of deaths from cardiovascular disease, type 2 diabetes, and cancer.[23] The estimated years of life lost was 6.5 for individuals with a BMI of between 40.0 and 44.9 and more than doubled to 13.7 years lost for individuals with a BMI of between 55.0 and 59.9.

Up until 2017, life expectancy in the U.S. had been on the rise, although the rate was slow. In 2018, the National Center for Health Statistics reported that life expectancy had, in fact, decreased for the first time by one-tenth of a year to 78.6 years. Whether this trend will continue is unclear, but what is crystal clear is that seventy-eight-plus years is a long time. And if a large portion of those years are spent as obese, the risk of developing an early comorbidity—the presence of two chronic diseases or conditions at the same time—is elevated.

---

23   Cari M. Kitahara et al., "Association between class III obesity (BMI of 40-59 kg/m2) and mortality: a pooled analysis of 20 prospective studies," *PLOS Medicine* 11, no.7 (July 2014): e1001673.

The 15 Leading Causes of Death in 2016

1. Heart disease
2. Malignant cancer
3. Accidents / unintentional injuries
4. Chronic lower respiratory diseases
5. Cerebrovascular diseases / stroke
6. Alzheimer's disease
7. Diabetes
8. Influenza and pneumonia
9. Kidney disease
10. Suicide
11. Sepsis
12. Chronic liver disease and cirrhosis
13. Hypertension and hypertensive renal disease
14. Parkinson's disease
15. Pneumonitis due to solids and liquids

Obesity & Type 2 Diabetes

The development of type 2 diabetes is closely linked to being obese, hence the term "diabesity" (diabetes + obesity). Forty years ago, diabesity wasn't even a real word, but since medical professionals began noticing the clinical association between obesity and type 2 diabetes, the term was coined. Forty years ago, type 2 diabetes wasn't at epidemic proportions either, but changes in lifestyle and nutrition have created a new health reality for 9.4% of the U.S. population (30.3 million people).[24] Although the rate at which newly diagnosed adult cases has decreased from 2008 to 2015, the total number of existing cases plus new cases has gone up annually. In 2015, the

---

24   Centers for Disease Control and Prevention, *Diabetes Report Card 2017*, (Atlanta, GA: Centers for Disease Control and Prevention, US Department of Health and Human Services, 2018), Online PDF.

year for which current statistics are available, approximately 1.4 million people ages 18 to 79 were newly diagnosed with type 2 diabetes.

By comparison, in 1958 about a half a million Americans, or 1% of the population, had type 2 diabetes.[25] *So, how did we get here from there—from 1% to 9.4%?* Let's take a look at nutrition from the standpoint of where our calories come from today. Food is readily available, and cheap calories (a.k.a. junk food and fast food) are relatively abundant. There's very little effort required to obtain this food, which complements, or enables, our sedentary lifestyle quite nicely. Modern conveniences like pizza delivery and drive-through fast food restaurants have an unanticipated flaw, however. Remember those hunter/gatherer ancestors? Well, they developed a survival mechanism by which their bodies stored excess calories as body fat to carry them from bountiful food times through lean times when food was scarce. This survival mechanism remains with us today.

Treating Obesity

Losing weight has a remarkable series of medical "side effects" that go well beyond simple aesthetics. Weight loss treats insulin resistance, pre-diabetes, and type 2 diabetes, as well as hypertension in some people. Multiple studies have shown that a 5 to 10 percent loss of body weight has been shown to improve insulin sensitivity, decrease fasting blood glucose levels, and reduce or eliminate the need for some diabetes medications.[26] In other words, losing weight can put type 2 diabetes into remission or even prevent it from developing in the first place. My caveat is, however, that the 5 to 10 percent weight loss should be **fat** loss, not muscle loss. Maintaining muscle tissue through exercise (BioEnergetic Element #3) is essential to maintaining a high basal metabolic rate so the body burns more calories at rest. Changing dietary habits is equally important, and I'll discuss some popular eating styles ("diets") later in this chapter.

---

25   Centers for Disease Control and Prevention, *Long-term Trends in Diabetes April 2017*, Online PDF.

26   Donna H. Ryan and Sarah Ryan Yockey, "Weight Loss and Improvement in Comorbidity: Differences at 5%, 10%, 15%, and Over," *Current Obesity Reports* 6, no.2 (June 2017):187-194.

Failures of the Food Pyramid

Depending upon how old you are, nutrition would have been taught to you in a different way compared to today's youth—whether it was the Food Wheel (circa 1984), the Food Guide Pyramid (circa 1992), or MyPyramid (circa 2005).[27] Today, kids are taught using MyPlate, which was unveiled in 2011 by the U.S. Department of Agriculture (USDA). Each new iteration of the four food groups was supposed to promote healthy eating among Americans.

The Food Wheel and the Food Guide Pyramid influenced people's eating habits (including mine), and believe me, it was a carb lover's dream! Pasta, rice, and bread were good for you—six to eleven servings daily—and the government was saying it was OK. It was also a time when saturated fat was reviled for its purported connection to heart disease. The low-fat food craze spurned the addition of more sugar to processed foods just to make them taste good after the fat was removed. Store shelves were awash with low-fat breads, low-fat cookies, low-fat ice cream, and low-fat potato chips. And, of course, because it was "low-fat," that meant that you could eat more of it, or so we thought.

There was always a small contingency of doctors, nutritionists, and health-minded individuals who didn't jump on the fat-bashing bandwagon and instead, held firm to the conviction that **sugar**—not fat—was public enemy number one. By virtue of being low-fat, many foods didn't satisfy our hunger as the full-fat versions did. So instead of eating two regular cookies, we ate three, four, or more of the low-fat variety just to feel satisfied. Four cookies (or the whole box) raise blood glucose levels higher and require the pancreas to secrete more insulin than two full-fat cookies. The blood glucose spike, followed by a slump, is going to make you feel like you need a nap, or more cookies. And, being sedentary promotes all those additional sugar calories getting stored as fat. Since then, much of the low-fat-diet thinking has been debunked, and there's also some evidence

---

27 "A Brief History of USDA Food Guides," USDA ChooseMyPlate, November 30, 2018, www .choosemyplate.gov.

that the sugar and processed foods industries had a hand in promoting the obesity epidemic.

Poisoned Food

There's no real doubt that our quest to grow more food, food that looks pretty, and food that won't spoil easily, has been quite successful. But perhaps this efficiency has been achieved with unintended, unhealthy, and even deadly consequences. Pesticides, heavy metals, antibiotics, and preservatives showcase our intellectual and technical prowess, but at what cost? No one would willingly douse their salad with an endocrine disruptor or a known carcinogen, but that's exactly what happens on a daily basis—without our consent. The G.I. tract and gut microbiome are the front line of defense against these environmental toxins, but they too suffer damage. If our daily nutrition keeps our bodies in the Stress State, how can we break free and rid our tissues of the toxins that have accumulated over the years of unintentional ingestion? Let's examine a few of the more pervasive toxins in today's foods.

Glyphosate

This broad-spectrum herbicide is more commonly known by its trade name Roundup®, and its use is ubiquitous by U.S. farmers. It was discovered in 1970 by John E. Franz, a Monsanto chemist, and became available for agricultural use in 1974. It is currently used in 130 countries, although an increasing number of nations, including many in the European Union, have restricted or banned its use due to concerns about toxicity and potential carcinogenic effects. The International Agency for Research on Cancer (IARC), a division of the World Health Organization (WHO), asserted in its 2016 Monograph that glyphosate is probably carcinogenic to humans, and there is a specific link to non-Hodgkin lymphoma.[28] IARC's analysis

---

28 "IARC Monograph on Glyphosate," World Health Organization: International Agency for Research on Cancer, 2016, www.iarc.fr.

identified two likely mechanisms of action when people are exposed to glyphosate: (1) DNA damage in blood cells and (2) increased oxidative stress.

It has been difficult to quantify the direct effects of glyphosate in humans, especially since we are exposed to so many different herbicides and chemical toxins. Rodent models, however, suggest that exposure to glyphosate-based herbicides during development affects communication between neurons, alters behavior, and modulates the gut microbiome.[29] Research shows that "safe" levels of glyphosate exposure can modify the gut microbiome before rats reach the comparable age to human puberty.[30] Mice that were chronically exposed to glyphosate developed anxious and depressive behaviors; analysis of their microbiome showed both a decrease in the number of key microbes and a decrease in the overall diversity of key microbes.[31] Even honey bees exposed to glyphosate experience unfavorable changes to the good gut bacteria, potentially harming their health.[32,33] Like humans, bees in a Stress State can suffer from compromised pollinating abilities, which may, in turn, affect our food supply.

In the last five or so years, the gut microbiome has been of increasing interest to researchers and medical practitioners for its influence on both physical and mental health. As we learn more, I believe this is where we will discover the "fix" for much of what ails us (more on this later). Glyphosate's primary action on weeds at the molecular level entails inhibiting a plant enzyme necessary for the synthesis of tyrosine, tryptophan, and

---

29 Julie Dechartres et al., "Glyphosate and Glyphosate-based herbicide exposure during the peripartum period affects maternal brain plasticity, maternal behavior and microbiome," *Journal of Neuroendocrinology* 31, no.9 (September 2019): e12731.

30 Quixing Mao et al., "The Ramazzini Institute 13-week pilot study on glyphosate and Roundup administered at human-equivalent dose to Sprague Dawley rats: effects on the microbiome," *Environmental Health* 17, no.1, (May 29, 2018): 50.

31 Yassine Aitbali et al., "Glyphosate based- herbicide exposure affects gut microbiota, anxiety and depression-like behaviors in mice," *Neurotoxicology and Teratology* 67 (May – June 2018): 44-49.

32 Erick V. S. Motta, Kasie Raymann, and Nancy A. Moran, "Glyphosate perturbs the gut microbiota of honey bees," *Proceedings of the Natural Academy of Sciences of the United States of America* 115, no.41 (October 2018): 10305-10310.

33 Nicholas Blot et al., "Glyphosate, but not its metabolite AMPA, alters the honeybee gut microbiota," *PLoS One* 14, no.4 (April 16, 2019): e0215466.

phenylalanine. It just so happens that these three amino acids are involved in the synthesis of neurotransmitters, hormones, and proteins. If we think of gut bacteria like "weeds," then glyphosate upsets the natural balance by reducing microbial diversity and abundance, thereby depleting the very microorganisms that produce what our bodies need to function optimally. It's definitely food for thought, and the coming years are likely to reveal irrefutable evidence of glyphosate's deleterious impact on human health. *But why wait?* Aim for organic produce as much as your budget permits.

Pesticides

The term *pesticide* includes chemicals that kill weeds (herbicide), fungus (fungicide), insects (insecticide), and rodents (rodenticide), though many people only think of the insecticide variety when they think of pesticides. And like the pests they aim to combat, pesticides come in a wide variety, and although there's far less agreement as to their individual connection to specific diseases, one thing is certainly clear: Just about every human being on planet Earth has been exposed to pesticides from the foods they eat. Pesticide residues can remain on fruits, vegetables, and grains but diminish significantly after harvest, when exposed to light, and when they are washed and cooked. The U.S. Environmental Protection Agency (EPA) sets safety standards for the allowable amount of pesticide residues on food that have a "reasonable certainty of no harm."[34] Now, I don't want anyone thinking, nor do I believe that consumers believe that pesticide use is risk-free. By their very nature, pesticides are intended to kill pests—hopefully, not humans—but some are more susceptible/sensitive to their effects and more so with repeated exposure.

Pesticides tend to drift when sprayed aerially, so produce from an organic farm may test positive for pesticides just because of its proximity to a conventional farm. Also, water run-off from pesticide-sprayed crops and contaminated rain can travel miles from the original source and show

---

34 "Regulation of Pesticide Residues on Food," EPA, Environmental Protection Agency, April 30, 2019, www.epa.gov.

up on organic farms. Conventional produce is 2.9 to 4.8 times as likely to contain pesticide residues as organic produce (as you might expect), but data from the USDA Pesticide Data Program (PDP) showed that 23% of the organic produce they sampled tested positive.[35] The Environmental Working Group (EWG)—you may know them as the creators of the "Dirty Dozen™"—developed an annual list of conventionally-grown vegetables and fruits with the highest likelihood of pesticide residues.[36]

2019 Dirty Dozen™

1. Strawberries
2. Spinach
3. Kale
4. Nectarines
5. Apples
6. Grapes
7. Peaches
8. Cherries
9. Pears
10. Tomatoes
11. Celery
12. Potatoes

Although not completely conclusive, research has demonstrated a connection between pesticide use—the toxicity of the ingredients and level of exposure—and asthma, type 2 diabetes, cancer, leukemia, and Parkinson's

---

35 Carl K. Winter and Josh M. Katz, "Dietary exposure to pesticide residues from commodities alleged to contain the highest contamination levels," *Journal of Toxicology* (May 15, 2011).

36 Environmental Working Group, "Dirty Dozen™ Fruits and Vegetables with the Most Pesticides," EWG's 2019 Shopper's Guide to Pesticides in Produce, www.ewg.org.

disease.[37] People who are more susceptible to these health risks include children, pregnant women and their unborn babies, the elderly, people who are immune-compromised, and those who have a genetic susceptibility to pesticide-linked diseases. The male reproductive system is also affected: sperm count, motility, and viability decrease; regeneration of new sperm is inhibited; and sperm DNA can be damaged. This leads to decreasing fertility rates and genetic defects in one's offspring.

The best course of action for all of us is to take some sensible precautions when selecting and preparing food. Fruits and vegetables should be washed with a vegetable brush under running water to remove any residue. Wax treated fruits (e.g., apples) may trap the residue between the skin and the wax, so peel and discard the skin. Peeling the skin off fruits and vegetables, in general, is a good idea. Again, if your budget permits, buy organically grown produce or try growing your own. You may be surprised just how different (and delicious) these taste compared to conventionally grown produce. Certainly, if you and your partner are having difficulties becoming pregnant—after ruling out any medical conditions—a good first step would be to go organic and eliminate pesticides in your immediate environment.

Antibiotics

Oral antibiotics are wonderfully effective when you have a bacterial infection, such as an upper respiratory infection, a sinus infection, or a urinary tract infection. They kill the "bad" bacteria that causes these types of infections, but you probably already know that they kill the "good" bacteria as well. It's why doctors like me recommend eating yogurt, kefir, and fermented vegetables after patients have completed a course of antibiotics—to help re-establish the good bacteria colonies in the gut microbiome. It's also why we don't prescribe antibiotics unless patients absolutely need them; we don't want them to develop antibiotic-resistant bacteria strains ("superbugs"). Even if you rarely need antibiotics and you're committed to

---

37 Ki-Hyun Kim, Ehsanul Kabir, and Shamin Ara Jahan, "Exposure to pesticides and the associated human health effects," *Science of the Total Environment* (January 1, 2017): 525-535.

avoiding antibiotics like the plague, eating a hamburger or a grilled chicken breast could very well be a daily assault on your gut microbiome.

Prior to 2017 in the U.S., it was legal to routinely provide antibiotics to commercially raised beef, pork, and poultry for the purpose of promoting rapid growth and curtailing bacterial infections, regardless of whether the animals were actually sick. Because livestock on large-scale commercial farms are generally raised in confined spaces, they are prone to bacterial infections that can spread quickly among their pen-mates. Today, antibiotics can be administered as both treatment and prevention to curtail an infection outbreak. To minimize the risk of antibiotic residues in meat, milk, and eggs, a withdrawal or washout period must be adhered to before the animal(s) can be slaughtered. The Centers for Disease Control and Prevention (CDC), Food and Drug Administration (FDA), and U.S. Department of Agriculture (USDA) promote this safeguard, but ultimately, it is up to the farmer to respect it. Unfortunately, the promise of profit may threaten the aspiration of public safety. Additionally, the increasing demand for animal protein in developing countries may outweigh public safety concerns and eventually lead to health problems, which regulations in developed countries seek to avoid.[38]

Low levels of antibiotic residues in food could lead to changes in the bacteria comprising the gut microbiome—either in numbers or diversity. This can lead to disease or development of antibiotic-resistant bacteria strains, in the same manner as prescription antibiotics.[39] You've probably heard the saying, "you are what you eat," but more realistically, it's "you are what they ate." And it's possible they just ate a whole lot of antibiotics or pesticides. So, ensure the safety of the food you eat, look for meat that is labeled "raised without antibiotics" or seek out pasture-raised or grass-fed meats at a specialty meat market or your local farmer's market.

---

38   Christy Manyi-Loh et al., "Antibiotic Use in Agriculture and Its Consequential Resistance in Environmental Sources: Potential Public Health Implications," *Molecules* 23, no.4 (March 30, 2018): pii: E795.

39   Zeuko'o Elisabeth Menkem et al., "Antibiotic residues in food animals: Public health concern," *Acta Ecologica Sinica* 39, no. 5, (November 20, 2018): 411-415.

Toxic Heavy Metals

You may have heard about toxic heavy metals or heavy metal poisoning, but a lot of people don't know what exactly these are and the impacts they have on our health. By definition, a toxic heavy metal is a dense metal or metalloid found naturally in the earth that can potentially be toxic, especially when it becomes concentrated. The most common and concerning heavy metals include arsenic, cadmium, chromium, lead, and mercury. Heavy metals can be absorbed by plants through the soil; by animals through their feed and the air they breathe; and by large fish who consume great quantities of smaller, contaminated fish who themselves consumed contaminated plankton. In turn, humans absorb heavy metals from plant, animal, and fish food sources, as well as inhaling or touching heavy metals. Once absorbed into human tissues, heavy metals can bind to structural proteins (e.g., collagen, elastin, keratin), enzymes, and nucleic acids (i.e., DNA, RNA) and interfere with their functioning within the human body. Long-term exposure or high-dose exposure can precipitate various forms of cancer, nervous system damage, diabetes, tissue damage, and brain disorders (see chart on the next page).

When it comes to nutrition, we're in a bit of a quandary. For years we've been telling patients that fish is good for them, but we now must reckon with the possibility that the presence of mercury in fish may compromise its overall health benefits. Fish in general is high in protein, vitamins B-12 and D, and iron and is a good source of iodine, selenium, and zinc. Fatty fish, such as salmon, trout, mackerel, and sardines, are high in two beneficial omega-3s—DHA (docosahexaenoic acid) and EPA (eicosapentaenoic acid)—which are beneficial for heart health.

So, like most things in life, *moderation* is key. Avoid ocean fish and seafood higher up on the food chain that contain higher levels of mercury. River and lake fish can also contain heavy metals, pesticides, and other contaminants if they are subject to local runoff from mining operations, coal plants, chemical manufacturing plants, and large-scale farming operations. Some physicians are recommending against fish in general and

75

Heavy Metal	Acute Exposure (a day or less)	Chronic Exposure (months or years)
Arsenic	Nausea Vomiting Diarrhea Encephalopathy Multi-organ effects Arrhythmia Neuropathy	Diabetes Hypopigmentation/ hyperkeratosis Cancer
Cadmium	Pneumonitis (lung inflammation)	Lung cancer Osteomalacia (softening of bones) Proteinuria (excess protein in urine; possible kidney damage)
Chromium	Gastrointestinal hemorrhage (bleeding) Hemolysis (red blood cell destruction) Acute renal failure	Pulmonary fibrosis (lung scarring) Lung cancer
Lead	Encephalopathy (brain dysfunction) Nausea Vomiting	Anemia Encephalopathy Foot drop/wrist drop (palsy) Nephropathy (kidney disease)
Mercury	Diarrhea Fever Vomiting	Stomatitis (inflammation of gums and mouth) Nausea Nephrotic syndrome (nonspecific kidney disorder) Neurasthenia (neurotic disorder) Parageusia (metallic taste) Pink disease (pain and pink discoloration of hands and feet) Tremors

against specific varieties—shark, swordfish, king mackerel, bluefin tuna—to women of childbearing age, pregnant women, breastfeeding mothers, or young children.[40] Others recommend no more than two to three servings of fish per week, preferably the ones with the lowest mercury levels based on the FDA/EPA guidelines for pregnant women and children.[41] A further delineation of healthy fish choices is SMASH—which stands for sardines, mackerel, anchovies, wild-caught salmon, and herring—which are small, oily fish that live in more remote, colder, and less polluted areas of the ocean.

As for the heavy metal content of fruits and vegetables, it's determined by the soil in which it was planted. If the soil is heavily contaminated, you could reasonably expect that your produce would have higher levels. So, unless you know exactly where your produce comes from and that soil has been tested and results publicly disclosed, you may never know for certain. But, because produce has high nutritional value (antioxidants, fiber, vitamins, minerals), the benefits probably outweigh the risks. The general rule is that leafy green vegetables and root/tuber vegetables accumulate heavy metals at a greater concentration than either fruits or grains, especially if they are cultivated with wastewater and/or are grown in contaminated soil.

Chemical Food Preservatives

Unprocessed whole foods have a very limited shelf life, so in order to extend their usability window, chemicals are applied. There are a variety of chemicals used in food preservation, which elicit harmful effects. People who are body-aware or do not generally consume preservatives may notice these effects sooner than people who have become desensitized. Here's a list of the most commonly used chemical preservatives:[42]

---

40 Tatiana Kimáková et al., "Fish and fish products as risk factors of mercury exposure," *Annals of Agricultural and Environmental Medicine* 25, no.3, (September 25, 2018): 488-493.

41 "Questions & Answers from the FDA/EPA Advice on Eating Fish," U.S. Food and Drug Administration, www.fda.gov.

42 Sanjay Sharma, "Food Preservatives and their harmful effects," *International Journal of Scientific and Research Publications* 5, no.4 (April 2015).

- **Sulfites:** Used in dried fruits and wine. Side effects include allergies, headaches, heart palpitations, and cancer. Example: sulfur dioxide.

- **Nitrates & nitrites:** Used to cure meats and processed meat products. Side effects: believed to cause stomach cancer. Example: sodium nitrite.

- **Benzoates:** Used to inhibit bacteria, mold, insects, or other micro-organisms from growing in foods (antimicrobial preservative). Side effects: allergies, asthma, and skin rashes; suspected role in brain damage. Examples: sodium benzoate, benzoic acid.

- **Sorbates/sorbic acid:** Used as an antimicrobial preservative in foods. Side effects (rare): hives and contact dermatitis. Examples: sodium sorbate, potassium sorbate.

The above list is not a comprehensive list, just some of the more prevalent worst offenders. In general, avoid foods designed to last a long time. When buying packaged foods, if you can't recognize all the ingredients on the label, put it back on the shelf. And don't forget, sugar and salt are also considered preservatives, although not of chemical origins.

Time to Reevaluate

Whew! I hope you haven't decided to give up on eating altogether now that you know there's quite a lot of potential hazards in our food supply. Being educated is half the battle. The other half is making healthier food choices based on what you just learned and continue to learn by being an informed consumer. Shop wisely for foods that enhance your health (e.g., fresh foods in their natural or "whole" state), not detract from it (e.g., processed foods). One of the easiest ways of doing this is to shop the outer perimeter of your grocery store; that's where the fresh fruits, vegetables, and meats are located. Pass up the middle aisles where all the high-sugar, processed, and well-preserved foods are located. Aim for organic, grass-fed, and pasture-raised if you can.

On to More Positive Things...

"In the morning, look at the glowing sunlight
and allow it to brighten the consciousness of your mind."
—Debasish Mridha

I consider sunlight a nutrient, and what could be more invigorating than warm sunlight shining upon your face? Stimulating your senses, your body, and your mind...welcoming you to a new day. Exposing yourself to sunlight is making a comeback as a biohack. The avoid-the-sun-at-all-costs, slather-on-the-SPF-100 folks (including most dermatologists) are getting some pushback from science and common sense. If you recall high school science, sunlight is the basis of life—via photosynthesis—on planet Earth; chloroplasts convert solar energy to chemical energy, which is necessary for glucose production so plants can grow and thrive. Animals consume plants for energy and nutrition to grow their muscle tissue, and then humans come along and eat a steak and a salad. The sun provides us with so much more than just food to survive. It is itself a nutrient that we should strive to attain daily for optimal health.

Without sunlight, the human body cannot manufacture the vitamin D it requires for a variety of metabolic functions. The ultraviolet rays hit the skin, thereby initiating vitamin D synthesis. Vitamin D is inert at this point, but becomes biologically active after two metabolic reactions: first, the liver converts vitamin D to 25-hydroxyvitamin D [25(OH)D], or calcidiol; and second, the kidneys convert calcidiol to 1,25-dihydroxyvitamin D [1,25(OH)$_2$D], or calcitriol. We commonly associate calcium with bone metabolism and as a means to prevent osteoporosis, but it is the vitamin D that promotes calcium absorption in the gastrointestinal tract so that it will be deposited in the bones; individuals with long-term insufficient vitamin D intake and/or sunlight exposure can develop thin or brittle bones.

Virtually every cell in the body has vitamin D receptors on it, which demonstrates the far-reaching impact vitamin D has in the body's overall functioning—from cell growth, to immune function, to neuromuscular function, to inflammation reduction.[43] Low vitamin D levels have been linked to an increased risk of premature (earlier than age 50) coronary artery disease (CAD), and the greater the vitamin D deficiency, the more extensive CAD.[44] Vitamin D deficiency is linked to hypertension and resistant hypertension (uncontrolled with three medications, or controlled with four or more medications).[45] Since so many chronic diseases are connected to an overactive immune system, getting sufficient vitamin D from sunlight could be a game changer.

And, as discussed in Chapter 2: SLEEP, morning sunlight plays an important role in regulating circadian rhythm so you get a better night's sleep. Sunlight increases serotonin production, which, in turn, contributes to your feelings of happiness and general well-being. At the same time, it decreases the risk of insomnia, depression, and Seasonal Affective Disorder (SAD), especially if where you live gets very little sunlight during the winter months.

Hopefully, all this wonderful news about sunlight and vitamin D will allay your fears about the dangers of the sun you've been warned about your entire life. Too much sun exposure can cause premature skin aging (wrinkles...ugh), so it's wise to cover up the areas you want to remain youthful looking—face, neck, and hands. Wear a wide-brimmed hat and cover your hands and arms with clothing. Expose the larger areas—torso and legs—and let them be your vitamin D solar panels; more surface area absorbs more sunlight and synthesizes more vitamin D. Your body is like a vitamin D battery because it can store the excess vitamin D for days when you aren't in the sun. Make this your daily ritual during the summer months, and you'll store enough vitamin D to get you through the winter months.

---

43   "Vitamin D," U.S. Department of Health and Human Services, National Institutes of Health Office of Dietary Supplements, nih.gov.

44   Hamidreza Norouzi et al., "Association of vitamin D deficiency and premature coronary artery disease," *Caspian Journal of Internal Medicine*, 10, no.1 (Winter 2019): 80-85.

45   Shiran Alagacone et al., "The association between vitamin D deficiency and the risk of resistant hypertension," *Clinical and Experimental Hypertension* 42, no.2, (April 2019): 1-4.

I've told you about how poor nutrition and man-made chemicals contribute to diabesity and sub-optimal health. If you break from this nutritional downward spiral, you can escape the Stress State, and I want to show you in the next chapter how to put nutrition and smart food choices to work for your body and your better health. Feed your body what it needs, and it will help propel you into your Thrive State.

5 to Thrive

1. We've covered this before and repetition is the branding iron of knowledge. We are our habits. We created them, so we can break them. We can also establish new ones. Remember, start with a tiny habit change. With the confidence that comes from breaking a single simple bad habit comes the motivation to establish new healthy ones. It's the stacking of healthy habits that will get you into the Thrive State.

2. The traditional food pyramid is outdated and has contributed to our obesity and chronic disease epidemic.

3. Beware of the many poisons in your foods, including heavy metals, pesticides, herbicides, antibiotics, and preservatives. Organic produce is your safest bet, as we have yet to discover the long-term health effects of pesticides like glyphosate. Avoid foods with long ingredients lists and chemicals you don't recognize.

4. Fish is a heart-healthy food source, but it is important to balance the risks, such as mercury buildup, with the benefits of eating fish regularly. Aim for moderation and remember SMASH (sardines, mackerel, anchovies, wild-caught salmon, and herring).

5. Pasture-raised or grass-fed, grass-finished meats are generally void of antibiotics, have a much better nutrient profile, and are a lot less inflammatory than industrially raised meats.

CHAPTER 5

YOUR PERSONAL FOOD BLUEPRINT

Given how many books, television shows, and infomercials are dedicated to extolling the virtues of a specific diet or nutritional supplement, perhaps you won't be surprised to learn that I decided to dedicate more than one chapter to the BioEnergetic Element of Nutrition. My decision was driven not only by the importance of this BioEnergetic Element, but by the complexity that surrounds this element. Although the act of eating is simple, the science around it is anything but. Our clinical understanding of food, nutrition, metabolism, and weight loss is complex, if not downright confusing, in today's world.

You may have heard the saying: "It's the truth as we know it today." Nutritional science seems to be an ever-changing field, and even the experts have differing opinions on what you should eat and what you should avoid. Fad diets come and go. Everyone wants a magic pill for weight loss. Fat is good; then it's bad; now it's good again. Egg yolks will give you a heart attack. Diet soda is sugar-free, so drink to your heart's content. It makes you want to throw up your hands and put your face down into a heaping bowl of full-fat ice cream with gooey chocolate sauce, chopped nuts, and artificially sweetened, aerosol, fake whipped cream.

Nutrition, and by that, I mean what you put into your mouth, has a profound effect on whether your body and mind are thriving or stressing. It sounds rather simple, but actually knowing what you should eat and following through with good choices are not necessarily easy. As I discussed in the previous chapter, quite a lot of the food supply is poisoned to some degree, and you may have little control over that aspect. In this chapter, which still deals with the BioEnergetic element of Nutrition, I'm going to focus more on foods themselves with a modest assumption that they are of high quality (i.e., organic and "clean"). I'll help you think of foods in terms of: *If I put this into my body, will it help me thrive physically and mentally, or will it place undue stress on or compromise my optimal functioning? Is it premium, mid-grade, or regular, or is it like putting sugar in your gas tank?*— literally and figuratively. Getting to the Thrive State requires spending a little extra—effort, not necessarily money—on premium-grade fuel for your internal engine.

Dr. V's NUTRITION Rx: Nutrition is complex. Knowing what you put in your mouth, where it comes from, and how it impacts your health is critical.

Feeding Your Gut Bugs

When you eat, you're really feeding your gut microbiome—the complex ecosystem inhabiting your gastrointestinal tract. It's comprised of trillions of microorganisms, including bacteria, viruses, and fungi (yeasts), which coexist to regulate metabolism; communicate with other cells in the body; influence brain functioning; manufacture vitamins the body needs; and turn genes on and off. Our "gut bugs" outnumber our cells by a factor of ten, so for every one human cell, there are ten microorganisms. Now, if that didn't wow (or frighten) you, this will for sure: The microbiome's genetic material, or DNA, outnumbers human DNA by a factor of 100. Keeping our gut bugs happy and thriving within their ecosystem is key to achieving the Thrive State. And by the way, these little guys have a preference for plant-based fiber, even though they'll eat just about anything you feed them—even if it is that bowl of ice cream with gooey chocolate sauce, chopped nuts, and artificially sweetened, aerosol, fake whipped cream.

Many people regard the microbiome as an independent human organ, and some even call it the "second brain" because of its significant impact on brain health. This three- to five-pound organ—recognized in the late 1990s—may be responsible for the "gut feeling" you get in certain situations. Its direct connection to the brain comes via the vagus nerve, also called the pneumogastric nerve, or the tenth cranial nerve, which influences the heart, lungs, and gastrointestinal (G.I.) tract. The communication between the microbiome and the brain—the gut-brain axis—is a bidirectional network between the neurons that govern functioning of the G.I. tract and the neurons of the central nervous system.[46] In essence, it means that your brain can give instructions to your microbiome and your microbiome can give instructions to your brain. And it's a whole lot more than simply gut feelings; research reveals that their back-and-forth conversations affect mood, cognition, and mental health.[47,48]

The predominant role the gut microbiome plays is maintaining gastrointestinal homeostasis (balance), and it functions better with a high microbial diversity. When it's out of whack—more bad microorganisms than good microorganisms—this is known as *dysbiosis*, or imbalance. Dysbiosis correlates with chronic inflammation in the G.I. tract, which, if not addressed, contributes to the development of inflammatory bowel diseases such as celiac, Crohn's disease, and ulcerative colitis. Due to the gut-brain axis, individuals with dysbiosis are likely to develop neurodegenerative, neurodevelopmental, and psychiatric disorders.[49]

---

46 Christine Fülling, Timothy G. Dinan, and John F. Cryan, "Gut Microbe to Brain Signaling: What Happens in Vagus...," *Neuron* 101, no.6 (March 2019): 998-1002.

47 Jeremy Appleton, "The Gut-Brain Axis: Influence of Microbiota on Mood and Mental Health," *Integrative Medicine: A Clinician's Journal* 17, no.4 (August 2018): 28-32.

48 Ting-Ting Huang et al., "Current Understanding of Gut Microbiota in Mood Disorders: An Update of Human Studies," *Frontiers in Genetics* 10, no.98 (February 2019): 98.

49 Diana Serra, Leonor M. Almeida, and Teresa C. P. Dinis, "The Impact of Chronic Intestinal Inflammation on Brain Disorders: the Microbiota-Gut-Brain Axis," *Molecular Neurobiology*, (April 3, 2019).

The goal of any diet or nutritional intervention should be directed, at least in part, to keeping the microbiome in a homeostatic state while encouraging high microbial diversity. Likewise, the body functions at peak levels when it is in homeostasis. Getting to your Thrive State should begin with a solid nutritional foundation that feeds, nourishes, and keeps your gut bugs happy. Achieving higher microbial diversity can be accomplished by eating a wide variety of foods, including prebiotics and probiotic-rich foods.

> **Dr. V's NUTRITION Rx:** You're never eating for just one; you're eating for the trillions of microorganisms inhabiting your gut microbiome. Feed them the best and cleanest you can afford.

The Leaky Gut Connection

"Leaky gut" is the lay term for what we doctors call increased intestinal permeability. It's an exceedingly common condition in which the delicate lining of the small intestine becomes more permeable than what is considered normal. The tight junctions between the cells comprising the gut lining normally keep the barrier between the gut and the bloodstream strong so that nothing gets through. If you have a leaky gut, the tight junctions loosen a bit, which allows microbes, toxins, and microscopic undigested food particles to pass right into the bloodstream. Once these substances get into the bloodstream, the immune system says, "Hey, I don't recognize these guys. They must be foreign invaders." And so, the immune system goes about initiating an inflammatory response to isolate and destroy the substances that should, rightly so, not be in the bloodstream. If the gut lining remains porous, the inflammation is ongoing, and this may eventually lead to the immune system losing its ability to distinguish between true foreign invaders (i.e., pathogens) and its own tissues—destroying them both.

Leaky gut is believed to be a consequence of our modern lifestyles—gut-irritating pharmaceutical drugs, acid-blocking medications, over-the-counter and prescription pain medications, antibiotic overuse and misuse, pesticide-contaminated foods, GMO foods, processed foods, and lack of or insufficient breastfeeding. It's a daily assault on the gut lining, not to mention the inhabitants of the G.I. tract—the microbiome—which depend on us for survival.

Some in the medical field remain skeptical about leaky gut, sometimes referred to as leaky gut syndrome. Nonetheless, and regardless of whether you call it leaky gut or increased intestinal permeability, evidence of it can be measured in urine or stool. In 2000, Alessio Fasano and his research team at the University of Maryland School of Medicine discovered the protein zonulin which modulates tight junction permeability.[50] Dr. Fasano's research continues to make strides in solidifying the connection between intestinal barrier function (tight junctions) and the onset of inflammation, autoimmunity, and cancer.

A healthy, strong, and non-porous gut barrier is important to immune health since approximately 70 to 80 percent of our immune system resides within the G.I. track. If three-quarters of immune function is in the gut, then the health of the gut microbiome itself is critical. This is also a reason that babies born vaginally tend to be healthier than babies born via Cesarean section. A vaginal birth exposes the newborn to Mom's diverse bacteria as he or she passes through the birth canal. The newborn's own G.I. tract is initially seeded with bacteria as the baby swallows and breathes in vaginal secretions. Additional bacteria transfer (and thus, immunity) occurs with breastfeeding.[51] Because a newborn's gut is considered immature, or not completely developed, it's naturally "leaky," and that's perfectly OK for a newborn. Mom's colostrum, which is expressed in the first 72 hours or so, helps seal up the microscopic holes between the tight junctions.

Prebiotics vs. Probiotics

These two terms sound familiar and can often be confusing, but, in fact, they're very different from each other, although one is necessary to feed the

---

50   Alessio Fasano, "Zonulin and Its Regulation of Intestinal Barrier Function: The Biological Door to Inflammation, Autoimmunity, and Cancer," *Physiological Reviews* 91, no.1 (January 2011): 151-75.

51   Amadou Togo et al., "Repertoire of human breast and milk microbiota: a systematic review," *Future Microbiology* 14, no.7 (May 2019): 623-641.

other. This may sound like an ancient Greek riddle, and surprisingly just as simple. Prebiotics are non-digestible fiber compounds (inulin) found in vegetables and fruits that promote the growth of beneficial bacteria in the large bowel. The top 10 prebiotic foods with the highest fiber content by weight include raw chicory root, raw Jerusalem artichoke, raw dandelion greens, raw garlic, raw leeks, raw onion, raw asparagus, raw wheat bran, cooked wheat flour, and raw bananas.[52] These non-living substrates, or foods, help the microbiome's existing probiotics—living microorganisms—grow, colonize, and essentially, crowd out the pathogenic bacteria. Typically, food-based probiotics are strains of bacteria or fermented yeast that are introduced into foods (e.g., yogurt, kefir, sauerkraut, pickled vegetables or fruits, miso soup, kimchi, and tempeh).

Many people, including me, take probiotic supplements—live bacteria strains in capsules. The usefulness and safety of probiotic supplements is not without scientific debate. A 2018 study showed that many probiotic strains simply pass through the body without colonizing.[53] However, as microbiome expert Lucy Mailing PhD suggests, although some probiotics may not colonize the gut, they still have beneficial effects in transit, including modifying gene expression, aiding in eating and digestion, and stimulating the immune system. Check with your doctor on which probiotic is right for you; I personally use and recommend MegaSporeBiotic from Microbiome Labs.

Nutrigenomics... Another Piece of the Nutrition Puzzle

Nutrigenomics—the study of the interaction between genes and nutrition—is an early 20th-century concept that takes on new significance in the era of obesity and chronic disease. Nutrigenomic researchers aim to understand the complex interactions between the microbiome's genetic makeup, metabolism, the immune system, and how nutritional intake

52   Alanna J. Moshfegh et al., "Presence of inulin and oligofructose in the diets of Americans," *The Journal of Nutrition* 129, no.7 (July 1999): 1407S-11S.

53   Niv Zmora et al., "Personalized Gut Mucosal Colonization Resistance to Empiric Probiotics Is Associated with Unique Host and Microbiome Features," *Cell* 174, no.6 (September 2018): 1388-1405.e21.

might modulate or influence these interactions. It's as complicated as humans are complicated beings. The specific application of nutrigenomics is to develop personalized nutrition intervention programs, which, when combined with lifestyle changes, can improve health across the board by treating or preventing chronic diseases.[54]

Because we all have a unique genetic make-up AND a unique microbiome, which has its own unique genetic make-up, there's no one-size-works-for-all diet, whether it be weight loss, weight maintenance, or weight gain. Two people can follow the exact same diet and have very different outcomes in terms of weight. Keep in mind that your ideal diet is influenced by the sum of the BioEnergetic Elements. Just think about these questions for a moment:

SLEEP:
- *Did you skimp on sleep, which led to two additional cups of coffee the next morning?*
- *Did you oversleep, which led you to skip breakfast so you wouldn't be late for work?*

EXERCISE/PHYSICAL ACTIVITY:
- *Do you prioritize regular exercise the same way you prioritize mealtimes?*
- *Is exercise a frequent excuse to eat junk food?*

STRESS:
- *Did a bad day at work cause you to eat an entire bag of potato chips?*
- *Do you eat a lot of sweets or carbs when you are sad or unhappy?*

MINDSET:
- *Do you refuse to try new vegetables because your parents made you eat all your vegetables as a youngster?*
- *Do you equate good behavior with sweets or desserts?*

---

54   John C Mathers, "Nutrigenomics in the modern era," *Proceedings of the Nutrition Society* 76, no.3 (August 2017): 265-275.

COMMUNITY/RELATIONSHIPS:

- *Does a successful personal relationship mean taking on the unhealthy eating habits of your partner?*
- *Do you enlist the help of people in your community when you're trying to eat healthy, or do you feel you have to go it alone?*

SPIRIT/PURPOSE:

- *Do you believe that your body—your temple—deserves premium or regular fuel?*
- *Do you eat to live, or live to eat?*

Before I get into a review of specific diets, I want to address the universal problem that people trying to lose weight have—sugar and carb addictions. It has only been recently in human history that refined sugars (sucrose, fructose, and most recently, high-fructose corn syrup) have become prevalent in most people's diets. The average American consumes 19 added teaspoons of sugar each and every day in foods and beverages such as sodas, coffee, energy drinks, fruit juices, cereals, granola bars, yogurt, candy, baked goods, and the like. Sugar can become addictive in the same way that cocaine can, and, in fact, research involving mice showed that sugar was *more* addictive.[55] The mice had a preference for sugar *over* cocaine. That's serious!

With sugar addiction, people lose control over their sugar and refined carbohydrate consumption, and that makes no one happier than the yeast living in and on the body. Yeast, such as *Candida albicans*, LOVE sugar because it helps them multiply and grow their colonies—in the mouth, G.I. tract, and genitals. When you get sugar cravings, it's as if the yeast cells are calling out to your brain, "Feed us. Now!" An overabundance of *Candida* can cause infections (genital yeast infection, oral thrush) or dysbiosis in the gut microbiome.

---

55   Magalie Lenoir et al., "Intense sweetness surpasses cocaine reward," *PLoS One* 2, no.8 (August 1, 2007): e698.

There are two main ways of tackling an addiction: (1) cold turkey and (2) slow turkey. If you choose door #2 (slow turkey), you need to be regimented and carefully pay attention to your sugar and simple/refined carbohydrate consumption so you will know that you are indeed doing a gradual step-down. Whether it's a reduction in total added sugars per day or eliminating a specific high-sugar food category one at a time, you want it to be something that you can live with so that you'll stick to it. Here are two examples, albeit over-simplified, but you get the idea.

EXAMPLE: **Reducing Total Daily Added Sugars**

Week #1: Reduce daily soda consumption from four 12-oz cans to three; cut the sugar in your coffee by one-third; limit yourself to two donuts instead of three.

Week #2: Reduce daily soda consumption from three 12-oz cans to two; cut the sugar in your coffee by half; limit yourself to one donut instead of two.

Week #3: Reduce daily soda consumption from two 12-oz cans to one; cut the sugar in your coffee by three-fourths; limit yourself to a half of a donut instead of a whole one.

Week#4: Don't drink any soda; drink your coffee black with no sugar (no artificial sweetener either); have a piece of fresh, organic fruit instead of a donut.

EXAMPLE: **Eliminating Specific High-Sugar Food Categories (Modified Cold Turkey)**

Week #1: Eliminate all sodas.

Week #2: Eliminate all sugar and artificial sweeteners from coffee, tea, and other beverages.

Week #3: Eliminate all baked sweets (pastries, donuts, cakes).

Week #4: Eliminate all other sources of added sugars in your diet.

On the other hand, some people will do better with door #1 (cold turkey); no doubt it can be tough, and you may be tempted to cheat, but about 30 days will get you past the sugar cravings. Try drinking a big glass of water or practice deep breathing for a count of 100 whenever a sugar craving strikes. In the end, you'll be happier and feel better because your blood glucose levels will remain more consistent over the course of the day. The *Candida* colonies will shrink to a manageable (homeostatic) level within the microbiome.

The Golden Rule of Healthy Eating

Eat foods that are organic, whole, minimally processed, GMO-free, and do not contain additives or preservatives.

Is the Right Diet for Me Out There?

If you're like most people trying to lose weight, you've probably tried several diets in your lifetime—with varying degrees of success. One of the biggest mistakes people make, in my opinion, is thinking of it as a "diet." The word simply has too much ugliness associated with it—deprivation, lack of self-control, isolation—so I prefer the term "modified eating style." Here are some traditional, trendy, environmentally conscious, and science-backed eating styles. Each has its own merits and drawbacks. I'll reveal my favorite at the end.

Vegetarian Eating Style

Vegetarians eliminate animal-sourced foods from their diets, including meat, poultry, fish, and seafood, generally based on ethical, cultural, religious, health-related, or economic motivations, or personal taste preferences. Plant-based foods are the mainstay of a vegetarian diet, including fruits, vegetables, roots, beans/legumes, grains, nuts, seeds, plant oils, and foods derived from plants (e.g., bread, pasta, tortillas). **Lacto-ovo-vegetarians** consume dairy products, such as milk, butter, yogurt, and cheese, as well as eggs. **Lacto-vegetarians** consume dairy products but avoid eggs. **Ovo-vegetarians** consume eggs but no dairy products. **Vegans**—true vegetarians in every sense of the word—avoid all food products that come from an animal, including eggs and dairy products. A vegan diet is naturally deficient in vitamin B$_{12}$ and does not provide enough omega-3 fatty acids, essential amino acids, vitamin D, and other important minerals. **Pescatarians**, who eat fish and seafood but not meat or poultry, often consider themselves predominantly vegetarian.

A common misconception is that vegetarians are skinny and lose weight easily because they don't consume high-fat meat and dairy products. But in reality, vegetarians are no more successful at losing weight than meat eaters. If you avoid meat but consume voluminous quantities of carbohydrates and sugar (and you're not swimmer Michael Phelps), you will gain weight. That's not to say that if you moderate your carb intake, avoid refined sugars, and eat more vegetables and fiber you can't lose or maintain a healthy body weight as a vegetarian.

Paleo Eating Style

The Paleo Diet, or Paleolithic Diet, is a high-protein, low-glycemic-load, dairy-free eating style popularized in the early 2000s by Loren Cordain, PhD Although not an original concept to Dr. Cordain, he does get a lot of the notoriety; his colleague Boyd Eaton is referred to as the father of the modern Paleo Diet movement. Paleo eating centers around the eating habits of our Paleolithic ancestors, which includes foods they obtained via hunting and gathering—vegetables, roots, fruits, nuts, and meat. Foods developed after the transition to an agricultural lifestyle—grains, legumes (e.g., beans, lentils, peanuts, soy), sugar, alcohol, coffee, salt, refined oils, dairy products, and processed foods—are excluded. Proponents of the Paleo Diet believe that human digestion today is essentially the same as it was during the 2.6-million-year-long Paleolithic era.

Nutrition proponents have put their own twist on the Paleo Diet, but any version that discourages salt consumption is close to the original. Dr. Cordain says his diet improves a person's energy levels throughout the day; blood lipid levels are improved; and sleep quality is improved, especially when individuals reduce or eliminate alcohol and salt.[56] Over time, body weight and composition are improved and some symptoms of illness and chronic disease may go away. Carbohydrates are allowed, but only those in the form of low-glycemic-index fruits and vegetables, which minimize blood glucose spikes and elevated insulin levels and decrease the risk of obesity, hypertension, abnormal cholesterol and blood lipids, and type 2 diabetes.

Primal Eating Style

The Primal Blueprint, written by Mark Sisson in 2009, began as a diet, but became more of a lifestyle since. The underlying premise is that we should be eating more like our ancestors did prior to the Industrial Revolution (though not as far back as the Paleolithic era). That is to say, without processed foods, sugar and artificial sweeteners, alcohol, refined vegetable oils (e.g., soybean and canola oils), grains, and legumes (e.g., beans, lentils, peanuts, soy). The rationale is that the human body did not adapt itself to these foods and was therefore never meant to consume them; this idea makes the Primal Diet a close cousin to the Paleo Diet, yet the one major difference is that Primal eating permits some dairy products. Consuming foods in their natural state or as close to natural as possible is encouraged. This includes vegetables, fruits, nuts, seeds, healthy fats (e.g., olive oil, avocado oil, coconut oil, butter), meats, fish, eggs, raw and fermented dairy products (e.g., raw milk, cheese, kefir), and natural sweeteners (i.e., raw honey, pure maple syrup). Preferred meat sources include wild game

---

56 Lauren Cordain, "Ten Questions about the Paleo Diet With Dr. Loren Cordain," The Paleo Diet®, January 4, 2020, thepaleodiet.com.

(e.g., deer, elk, venison), rather than beef; if you do eat beef, it should be grass-fed and organic. Fruits, vegetables, and eggs should also be organic. Remember, everything was organic prior to the Industrial Revolution.

For weight loss, the primal style of eating recommends strictly limiting carbohydrate consumption to between 50 and 100 grams per day. This entails reading food labels and knowing the carb content of fresh, whole foods. Periods of intermittent fasting (to be discussed a little later) can be utilized for quicker weight loss.

Keto Eating Style

The ketogenic (keto) diet is characterized by high-fat, low-carbohydrate, and adequate-protein intake and was developed in the 1920s as a medical treatment for epilepsy in children. The diet—70% fat, 20% protein, and 10% carbohydrates—stimulates the body to utilize fat for fuel rather than carbohydrates. Normally, the brain is fueled by glucose converted from carbohydrates, but with a keto diet, the liver converts fat into fatty acids and ketones. The keto diet has been shown to decrease the number of seizures by approximately half in half of children and young people.[57] Some adults with epilepsy benefit from the ketogenic diet, and there's an increasing body of research suggesting that people with brain disorders such as Alzheimer's disease, autism, and brain tumors can benefit as well.

Ketogenic diets have some fairly dramatic health benefits as a result of the body and brain switching from glucose as fuel to ketones: reduced abdominal (belly) fat; increased energy production; increased stem cell production; improved gene expression; improved immune function; decreased inflammation and oxidative stress; and improved cognitive functioning. These benefits are similar to severe calorie restriction diets which have been shown to increase lifespan in mice; mice on ketogenic diets also live longer without calorie restriction.[58] By converting the body from a

---

57   Eric H Kossoff and Huei-Shyong Wang, "Dietary therapies for epilepsy," *Journal of Biomedical Science* 36, no.1 (January – February 2013): 2-8.

58   Megan N. Roberts et al., "A ketogenic diet extends longevity and healthspan in adult mice," *Cell Metabolism* 5, no.26 (September 2017): 539-546.e5.

glucose-burning engine to a fat-burning engine, the body becomes more efficient at using its own fat as fuel, thus reducing obesity and abdominal fat in particular. Decreasing obesity is key to reducing the risk of type 2 diabetes, among other health conditions.

Even though ketones are thought of as "clean-burning" fuel and thus, a more preferred energy source, many people find it difficult to actually eat that much fat on a daily basis. Additionally, side effects of eating so little fiber include constipation and vitamin and mineral deficiencies. The Atkins Diet is based on ketogenic principles. Fortunately, there are two biohacks that provide similar health benefits and are much easier to achieve than getting your body into a long-term ketogenic state.

Biohack #1: Intermittent Fasting / Time-Restricted Eating
This entails fasting for a period of at least 14 to 16 hours every day—typically overnight, from after the dinner meal until the next morning's breakfast. You can think of it as a rest period so your body to repair itself, remove the day's metabolic waste from the body and brain, and stimulate the cell recycling process also known as autophagy. Because this rejuvenation process is so important to the Thrive State, it's critical that you get a good night's sleep.

Biohack #2: MCT Oil & Coconut Oil
This entails consuming MCT (medium-chain triglyceride) oil one or more times a day. Some people also add coconut oil at the same time as MCT for added benefit. The MCT oil produces ketones quickly, and coconut oil extends the body's ability to continue producing ketones throughout the day. Adding this mixture to hot coffee or tea makes it more palatable for most people (just avoid the sugar and artificial sweeteners). Be sure to use a high-quality MCT oil and virgin coconut oil. Substituting grass-fed butter or ghee for the coconut oil is also an option.

Medium Chain Triglycerides & MCT Oil

There are four types of medium chain triglycerides, also known as fatty acids. They are capronic acid (C6), caprylic acid (C8), capric acid (C10), and lauric acid (C12). Each MCT has unique health benefits, including increasing energy levels, boosting metabolism, and providing antimicrobial action.

MCT oil is a purified extract of coconut oil. Coconut oil contains healthy fats, including more than 50% MCTs, and when the MCTs are extracted and concentrated, MCT oil serves as a highly efficient fuel source. The MCTs go to the liver where they are metabolized and converted to energy. This process promotes fat burning through the production of ketones.

Intermittent Fasting Eating Style

Intermittent fasting isn't just a biohack; it's a stand-alone, science-backed eating style that serves a physiological purpose beyond weight loss and has its roots in many cultures and religions around the world. Aside from the duration and practice specifics, all fasts share a common goal of demonstrating personal sacrifice and cleansing. Ancient peoples who first began the practice of fasting may not have known its anti-aging value but were certainly healthier for doing it. Fast forward to the 21st century when Japanese cell biologist Yoshinori Ohsumi discovered the mechanisms of autophagy and won the 2016 Nobel Prize in Physiology or Medicine and the 2017 Breakthrough Prize in Life Sciences.

Autophagy (autophagocytosis) is the cell's natural "recycling" process that disassembles unnecessary or dysfunctional cellular debris (waste) and converts it into usable components to refuel the mitochondria and triggers stem cell generation. This cellular recycling cycle creates renewal and efficiency within the cells, and is believed to help the body defend against disease and aging.[59] In fact, non-efficient autophagy—the accumulation of cellular garbage—is hypothesized as one of the root causes of neuro-degenerative and inflammatory diseases. Non-efficient autophagy is akin to hoarding junk; it takes up space, fulfills no real purpose, and creates a health hazard, and thus needs to be cleaned out and recycled/repurposed. As one ages, the capacity for autophagy decreases and so does the immune system's ability to defend the body against illness and disease.

Intermittent fasting (IF) stimulates autophagy. The process of autophagy kicks in after about 16 hours of fasting, so the more time between the last meal of the day and the first meal of the following day, the better. When it's time to break the fast, utilize the MCT oil biohack, rather than eating a full breakfast. Cycles of IF can be incorporated into any eating style, and the fasting duration can be extended to two to three days. As the fast lengthens, the body begins to utilize stored fat for fuel, which precipitates weight loss. Generally, this would be a water-only fast, but not everyone can tolerate such a long time without food, and so, there are various iterations depending on the patient's goal.

> **Dr. V's NUTRITION Rx:** There's a time for cellular feeding and a time for cellular cleaning. Take care to do both efficiently for maximal health.

Fasting Mimicking Diets (FMD) can achieve the benefits of fasting without the "starvation" component. The ProLon 5-Day Fasting Mimicking Diet® initiates autophagy and stem cell generation while supplying sufficient food to maintain lean muscle mass (prolonfmd.com). The fast duration is only five days, but the program delivers the benefits of a longer fast while preventing the potential side effects of not eating. Patients participate in the ProLon 5-day fast once a month, or once every two to three months, and eat their normal healthy diet the other days —depending on their goals of either weight loss, cellular clean-up and rejuvenation, or both.

---

59 Noboru Mizushima and Masaaki Komatsu, "Autophagy: renovation of cells and tissues," *Cell* 147, no.4 (November 2011): 728-41.

Pegan Eating Style

The Pegan Diet was created in 2014 by Mark Hyman, MD and is a hybrid of the best features of paleo and vegan eating styles; it is detailed in his 2018 book, *FOOD: What the Heck Should I Eat?* Dr. Hyman recommends produce (plant fiber) represent about 75% of your plate—the main course. That's the vegan component. Grass-fed, sustainably raised meat should be a side dish or a condiment and no more than four to six ounces per meal. That's the paleo component. This hybrid model fixes the nutrient deficiencies of the vegan diet and removes the overused excuse to eat too much meat of the Paleo Diet.

Dr. Hyman based the Pegan Diet on his 30 years of experience with patients and sound nutritional science; it's not meant to be a diet but a lifestyle, and it's not all that difficult to follow. Personally, I'm a big proponent of Dr. Hyman's approach to healthy eating, and I recommend the pegan style eating as a way to reach your Thrive State. Intermittent fasting and the MCT oil/ coconut oil biohack fit easily into the Pegan Diet for stimulating weight loss. Dr. Hyman suggests 2-3 tablespoons of a 1:1 mix of MCT oil and coconut oil three times a day.

The 13 Pillars of the Pegan Diet:[60]

SUGAR: Avoid it in all its forms (fructose, high fructose corn syrup) and the foods which the body converts to "sugar"—refined carbohydrates and flour. It may be used as an occasional treat, but never let it become a significant part of your daily nutrition.

PLANT-BASED FOODS: Fill your plate with mostly non-starchy vegetables, especially the ones that are deeply colored. Choose a wide variety for nutrient diversity and to satisfy your microbiome. If you must eat starchy vegetables, select winter squash or sweet potatoes, and eat only one-half cup per day; avoid potatoes (that includes French fries!).

---

60   Mark Hyman, *FOOD: What the Heck Should I Eat?* (New York: Little, Brown and Company, 2018).

FRUITS: Eat low-glycemic fruits such as berries, kiwis, and watermelon. Higher glycemic fruits like grapes, cantaloupe, and honeydews should be eaten sparingly, and dried fruits should be regarded as a "treat."

CONTAMINANTS: Avoid foods that have been contaminated by pesticides, antibiotics, hormones, heavy metals, chemical additives, preservatives, dyes, artificial sweeteners, or have GMO (genetically modified organism) origins.

HEALTHY FATS: Eat omega-3 fatty acids and fat from healthy sources such as nuts, seeds, olive oil, avocados, and avocado oil. Saturated fats are OK as long as they're from sustainably harvested fish, grass-fed meats, grass-fed butter or ghee, organic virgin coconut oil or butter, and whole eggs.

UNHEALTHY OILS: Avoid vegetable oils commonly used for frying such as corn, canola, sunflower, soybean, and grapeseed. Definitely stay away from margarine and products with trans-fats. Cold-pressed nut and seed oils, such as walnut, macadamia, and sesame, should only be used in small quantities as a flavoring.

DAIRY: Dairy should be avoided by anyone who is lactose-sensitive but for others can be consumed in moderation if it is from an organic, grass-fed source, preferably goat or sheep. Yogurt and kefir are OK occasionally as long as they are not sweetened with sugar or artificial sweeteners.

MEAT & ANIMAL PRODUCTS: Grass-fed or pastured, sustainably raised meat should be a side dish with a serving size of no more than 4 to 6 ounces.

Meat: Friend or Foe?

Grass-fed or pasture-raised meats are nutritionally superior to conventionally raised meat for a few simple reasons. First, the nutritional content of beef, for example, is related to what the cows ate. "Happy" cows roaming around in the pasture eat grass (their natural diet), which contains more omega-3 fatty acids and conjugated linoleic acid and fewer omega-6 fatty acids which as a whole, contributes to less inflammation in the body. Omega-6s are pro-inflammatory and are much more predominant in grain-fed meats. Eating grass produces meat that contains important antioxidants, vitamins, and minerals, such as beta-carotene, glutathione, lutein, superoxide dismutase, zeaxanthin, B vitamins, vitamin E, iron, phosphorus, potassium, and zinc. Second, pasture-raised cows are less likely to contain antibiotic residues because they are generally healthy and don't require antibiotics. Also, conventionally raised beef is more likely to test positive for antibiotic resistant bacteria (MRSA) or E. coli. Lastly, pasture-raised animals develop naturally; they use their muscles to walk around freely, and farmers aren't trying to fatten them up with grains, so they're leaner.

FISH: Eat only low-mercury fish that is high in omega-3 fatty acids and sustainably raised or harvested; this includes wild-caught salmon, sardines, anchovies, and herring.

GLUTEN: Avoid gluten, especially if you are gluten-sensitive, or eat it only occasionally if you can tolerate it. Aim for an heirloom (non-GMO) wheat variety, such as einkorn.

GLUTEN-FREE WHOLE GRAINS: Eat these low-glycemic grains sparingly and only half a cup (cooked) per meal—amaranth, black rice, buckwheat, quinoa, and teff.

BEANS & LEGUMES: Avoid starchy beans as much as possible to prevent digestive problems and possible mineral absorption impairment. If you must satisfy a bean craving, lentils are best, and have only one-half cup (cooked) per day.

PERSONALIZED NUTRITION: Work with a functionally trained nutritionist or doctor to determine which types of food work best with your body and your microbiome. This "bio-individuality" approach will help ensure you achieve your optimal nutrition intake.

We've Come a Long Way, Baby!

Artificial Intelligence & Nutrition

Now that you have a fairly good understanding of nutrition as a BioEnergetic Element, I'll share with you the future of nutrigenomics. With help from artificial intelligence (A.I.), we have the capability of pinpointing exactly what foods and supplements your body and your gut microbiome need for optimal functioning. A.I. takes the guesswork out knowing which foods you should eat and which you should avoid, even when both choices are considered "healthy." There are many companies pushing the envelope of microbiome analysis and nutrigenomics, and one such company that has this incredible technology is called Viome (www.viome.com). Their tests can establish whether your microbiome is functioning optimally in a very granular way, so that you can take specific steps you know will be beneficial.

Becoming More Deliberate with Your Nutrition Choices

In this chapter especially, I have endeavored to explain to you the different types of diets and eating styles that revolve around different nutritional choices. You'll notice that I have refrained from telling you that you must adopt a certain diet, or that I endorse one particular diet above all others. That is because I don't believe in a one-size-fits-all approach to nutrition. There is no objective "best" diet for you; in fact, your personal "best" diet is to a certain extent highly dependent on your personal genetic and epigenetic makeup.

And so, I have refrained from giving you a simple "Dr. V gives his official stamp of approval to this particular diet" approach, but I do have a Thrive State Food Blueprint if you're looking for a solid place to start (see following figures). You should review these chapters and determine what works best

NON-STARCHY VEGETABLES

At least
1/2 of your plate

PROTEIN

Each protein serving
should be no larger
than your palm

STARCH

Limit if you're diabetic.
Starches can comprise
of 1/4 of plate depen-
ding on activity
levels and goals.

FOOD BLUEPRINT

COOKING IN WATER IS BEST

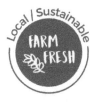

Local | Sustainable
FARM FRESH

Organic
ORGANIC FOOD

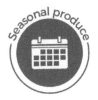

Seasonal produce

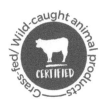

Grass-fed/ Wild-caught animal products
CERTIFIED

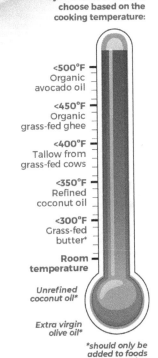

If you decide to use oils,
choose based on the
cooking temperature:

<500°F
Organic
avocado oil

<450°F
Organic
grass-fed ghee

<400°F
Tallow from
grass-fed cows

<350°F
Refined
coconut oil

<300°F
Grass-fed
butter*

**Room
temperature**

*Unrefined
coconut oil**

*Extra virgin
olive oil**

*should only be
added to foods
after cooking

103

FOOD BLUEPRINT

FAT
1-2 TBL
added to meals

SWEETENERS
Use sparingly!
• Stevia   • Monk fruit

FRUIT
~1 cup of berries
per day

HERBS/SPICES
Liberally added
to meals

DRINKS
• Plain filtered water (can
  add organic lemon/lime/
  mint), unsweetened
• Sparkling water with no
  added sweeteners
• Organic herbal teas

AVOID:

- Processed foods (anything that is in a package)
- Foods contaminated by pesticides, antibiotics, hormones, heavy metals, chemical additives, preservatives, dyes, and artificial sweeteners
- Alcohol, GMOs, Gluten
- Sugar (and all its forms including fructose and high-fructose corn syrup)
- Dairy should be avoided by anyone who is lactose sensitive but for others can be consumed in moderation if it is from an organic, grass-fed source, preferably goat or sheep
- Vegetable oils such as corn, canola, sunflower, palm/oil, corn oil, peanut oil, soybean, and grapeseed. Definitely stay away from margarine and products with trans-fats

FOOD BLUEPRINT

UNLIMITED
NON-STARCHY VEGETABLES

- Alfalfa sprouts
- Arugula
- Artichoke
- Asparagus
- Bamboo shoots
- Beans (green, Italian, yellow or wax)
- Bean sprouts
- Beets
- Bok choy
- Broccoli
- Brussels sprouts
- Cabbage
- Cauliflower
- Celery
- Chicory
- Chinese cabbage
- Chinese spinach
- Cucumber
- Eggplant
- Fennel

- Garlic
- Green onions
- Hearts of palm
- Herbs (parsley, cilantro, basil, rosemary, thyme, etc.)
- Jicama
- Kohlrabi
- Leeks
- Lettuce (endive, escarole, romaine or iceberg)
- Mushrooms
- Okra
- Onions
- Parsley
- Peppers (green, red, yellow, orange, jalapeño)
- Purslane
- Radishes
- Rapini
- Okra
- Onions

- Parsley
- Purslane
- Radishes
- Rapini
- Rhubarb
- Rutabaga
- Sauerkraut
- Scallions
- Shallots
- Snow peas or pea pods
- Spinach
- Summer squash
- Swiss chard
- Tomatillos
- Tomatos
- Turnips
- Water chestnuts
- Watercress
- Zucchini

STARCHES (Limit if diabetic)

- Sweet potatoes
- Beans, legumes, lentils
- Beets
- Carrots
- Green peas

- Parsnips
- Plantain
- Pumpkin
- Taro
- Squash

- Yams
- Quinoa
- Quinoa pasta

SPICES & HERBS

- Ginger
- Mint
- Oregano
- Thyme
- Rosemary

- Cinnamon
- Onion powder
- Garlic
- Parsley
- Black pepper

- Cilantro
- Cumin
- Cardamom
- Curry powder

* Any herbs that work well with your body can be used liberally

105

FOOD BLUEPRINT

HEALTHY OILS

- Olive oil
  (do not heat)
- Pumpkin seed oil
  (do not heat)
- Walnut oil
  (do not heat)
- Flaxseed oil
  (do not heat)
- Grass-fed butter (300F)

- Coconut oil
  (refined) (350F)
- Refined Sunflower oil
  (450F)
- Grass-fed ghee (450F)
- Grapeseed oil (485F)
- Avocado oil (520F)

*Oils to Avoid: Canola Oil, Vegetable Oil, Safflower Oil, Palm Oil/Shortening, Soybean Oil, Corn Oil, Peanut Oil

IDEAL SOURCES OF PROTEIN

- Grass-fed or pastured, sustainably raised meat or organ meats
- Organic, free range chicken and eggs
- Low-mercury, wild-caught fish. Remember SMASH (Sardines, Mackerel, Anchovies, Salmon, Herring). Also trout, haddock, and sole.
- Organic sprouted lentils, black beans, shelled hemp seeds, chia seeds

FLAVORING / CONDIMENTS

- Organic, raw, unsweetened cacao
- Vinegar
- Sea salt

- Himalayan sea salt
- Organic mustard
- Coconut aminos

HEALTHY FATS

- Avocado
- Olives
- Nuts
- Seeds

- Grass-fed butter or ghee
- Whole eggs
- Oils listed on the Healthy Oils list

106

for you. My recommendation is to try what I tried. Start with one specific, tangible change to your daily diet—a change that you can implement today, without needing to wait for the delivery of any weight-loss shakes or specialized nutrition plans. You can use the lessons of these chapters as inspiration for what change you choose to implement.

Do I Really Need to Supplement?

I often get asked if nutritional supplements are really a necessary part of Nutrition. The simple answer is YES. Since many people aren't following a traditional hunter-gatherer lifestyle, eating only wild plants, game, and fish, getting a lot of direct sunlight and exercise, sleeping well, and existing in a stress-free environment and because many of our soils are nutrient depleted and we are exposed to many environmental toxins, up to 90 percent of Americans are functionally deficient in micronutrients, vitamins, minerals, and fatty acids. Over time, these nutrient deficiencies lower your BioEnergetic State, make you more prone to chronic disease, including diabetes and cancer, and increase your susceptibility to infection, fatigue, depression, and other chronic symptoms of just not feeling well.

As a baseline rule for everyone, I recommend taking a high-quality multivitamin and high-quality purified fish oil (EPA/DHA). I also advocate for additional vitamin D3 and magnesium, as these are the most common nutritional deficiencies. Lastly, to support your mitochondria—your cells' energy centers—I also promote taking alpha-lipoic acid and CoQ10.

On top of the baseline recommendations, additional nutrients may be useful to support specific biological systems, defend against chronic disease states, and promote optimal desired performance. For example, because I once had diabetes, I use supplements that promote insulin sensitivity and healthy blood sugar levels, such as berberine, chromium, Ceylon cinnamon, and green tea catechins. Medicinal mushrooms, such as reishi, cordyceps, maitake, turkey tail, and lion's mane, as well as astragalus, beta glucans, and Vitamin C and D3 are excellent for immune system support. A functional or integrative doctor can help personalize a supplement regimen that works best for your lifestyle needs and health goals. Like me, they may also conduct a micronutrient test to check for specific micronutrient deficiencies.

One final note, it is important to be vigilant about the brands of supplements you take. The federal government doesn't regulate dietary supplements the same way as pharmaceuticals. With a poor-quality supplement, it's possible that the dosages don't match with the labels, the formulation may not be optimized for absorption, and the capsules may be filled with additives, colorings, and allergens. Some words to look out for on the manufacturer's label are "GMP certified," which means the company follows good manufacturing practices, and that supplements are "third party tested" to assure the purity of the supplement. In close, do some research about the brands before you buy and take recommendations from the experts you trust. For more recommendations on specific supplements, visit thrivestatebook. com/resources.

If You Don't Feel Great, ELIMINATE!

If you've followed the guidelines in the Thrive State Food Blueprint, and you're still experiencing symptoms like bloating, brain fog, poor sleep, poor digestion, skin rashes, mood issues, hormonal issues, joint pain, or other chronic symptoms on the "not feeling well" spectrum, it's possible you may have a food sensitivity. Food sensitivities might affect you immediately or they may take a few days, which can make it difficult to determine what foods might be causing various problems. If you think you may have a food sensitivity, talk to your doctor about an elimination diet protocol. Taking out specific trigger foods such as gluten, dairy, grains, sugar, alcohol, and caffeine for a duration of time is a way for your body to hit the reset button on your health. After following an elimination diet for a certain duration, you can then strategically add foods back in to see how you tolerate them.

The First Step Is the Simplest Step

Nutrition is a complex field. But that first step to strengthening this BioEnergetic Element can be very simple. For me, it was cutting out the sugary coffee drinks. Your first step can be just as simple... and just as significant.

My guess is, you are already evaluating which nutritional changes are right for you. For nutrition, there's no time like the present. Your one change that you make today could include switching to different fish dishes to avoid mercury, reducing your gluten intake, or eating more low-glycemic fruits.

As my own guide for you, I list the BioEnergetic Enhancers and Distractors for NUTRITION below.

	BioEnergetic Enhancers	BioEnergetic Disruptors
NUTRITION	– Organic, minimally processed – Sustainably raised meat – Clean drinking water – Good fats – Intermittent fasting	– Pesticides and other toxins – Factory-farmed meat – Polluted drinking water – Sugar, processed foods, bad oils

5 to Thrive

1. Your gut microbiome affects your brain health, immune health, psychological well-being, and likelihood to get chronic disease. Eating a wide variety of foods and probiotic-rich foods is essential for gut health.

2. Sugars and processed carbohydrates put your cells in the Stress/ Survive State and are the drivers of diabesity and many chronic diseases.

3. Fasting has anti-aging benefits because it stimulates autophagy (cell recycling). This process kicks in after about 16 hours of fasting.

4. There is no one-size-fits-all eating style; everyone's bodies are different and require different nutrient ratios depending on their lifestyles and health goals. Try adapting your diet with a simple change to start, such as cutting out sugar or processed foods. The Thrive State Food Blueprint is a great starting point. You can also visit thrivestatebook.com/resources for supplement recommendations.

5. Chronic symptoms like bloating, brain fog, poor sleep, poor digestion, skin rashes, mood issues, hormonal issues, and joint pain may be signs of a food sensitivity. Talk to your doctor about an elimination diet, which can help identify food sensitivities and reset your health.

To download a PDF copy of the Thrive State Food Blueprint and for additional resources on how to optimize nutrition, including supplements and other biohacks, visit thrivestatebook.com/resources.

CHAPTER 6

GETTING YOUR MOVE ON

At seven o'clock most mornings I usually can be found at the ETT Mecca, an exclusive gym in Hollywood. Until late 2022 you also would have found a very fit, very loud, very nice guy named Eric "The Trainer" Fleishman, cheerfully yelling at me. Eric, who passed away unexpectedly just before the release of this new edition, wasn't only my trainer; he was also a brother, mentor, and one of my biggest cheerleaders. Eric saw the best in people even before they saw it within themselves. I can't tell you the difference it made in my life to have someone believe in me that much. Our Thrive State, and our belief in others, is a penetrating force that can lift the spirit and hearts of all those around us. Eric's brilliant light will forever live within me. Rest in Power, brother.

It was usually me, Eric, and four or five others running—we call ourselves the WolfPack—through a series of exercises until we were sweaty, breathing heavily, and generally exhausted. Or, at least, I was.

This approach to MOVEMENT, the third Bioenergetic Element, works really well for me, and here's why. First, we are a small group of five regulars: my own miniature community of workout buddies. These are people I've come to respect and appreciate, and that means I want them to succeed, and they want me to succeed. We can push each other. I don't want to be the slacker in the group, but I also know everyone well enough that I won't be too embarrassed if I fall flat on my face.

Second, there's an atmosphere of positivity. And for that, I have to give a lot of credit to Eric. He was one of the most positive people I know. He was someone constantly breathing down my neck, stridently encouraging me to push myself harder... but he was awfully nice about it! And, crucially, I know myself well enough to know that I prize that positivity.

Third, I am a big believer in working out first thing in the morning. I begin my day by immediately elevating my Bioenergetic state. By the time the workday starts, I have given myself a burst of endorphins as well as a major accomplishment. I feel prepared for anything else the day throws my way because I have already pushed myself. I have reminded myself of what I can do if I put my mind to it. I feel capable of *responding* to a challenge rather than just *reacting* to it.

Finally—and perhaps most importantly—there is a sense of account-ability. I have a social obligation to show up to my morning exercises. My instructor is expecting me, as are my buddies. And sometimes, I need that push. After all, 7:00 a.m. can feel awfully early!

Look, I know that exercise is not always fun. Sometimes it feels like a chore. Sometimes we would rather do anything else. But we also know that if we want to thrive, we have to move our bodies. So, let's discuss what you should know about health, exercise, and how to lay the physical foundation for your Thrive State.

Stand Up for Your Health

BREAKING NEWS... Sitting is the new smoking! Maybe you've heard that a sedentary lifestyle is as unhealthy as smoking cigarettes. If you haven't, you'd better sit up (pun intended) and pay attention. Millions of Americans have given up smoking in the last few decades, much to the chagrin of the tobacco industry, but which industry profits when you take up sitting— chair manufacturers? Chronic sitting, as I like to call it, is an unfortunate consequence of our modern lifestyles. Whether it's sitting at a desk for eight hours at work, another hour or two in traffic, and all evening long in front of a computer screen, tablet, smartphone, or TV as we attempt to de-stress from all that sitting earlier in the day, it's far from what the human body was meant to be doing. You remember the old saying, "Use it or lose it"? Well, we're definitely losing something important—our health. So, this chapter is about the fourth BioEnergetic Element—MOVEMENT— to which I ask you to say with me right this moment, "Move it or lose it!"

Research, not to mention common sense, suggests that extended periods of sitting are related to bigger waistlines and rear-ends. No real surprise since less energy is expended while sitting than when you stand or move your body, and this can easily pack on the pounds. But, as I discussed in previous chapters, obesity is linked to a host of other unhealthy conditions that prevent you from thriving (e.g., hypertension, elevated blood glucose and cholesterol levels, and excess abdominal fat), thus contributing to type 2 diabetes, cardiovascular disease and cancer, which may ultimately increase your risk of premature death. A systematic review of the research published in 2015 in the *Annals of Internal Medicine* brought this ominous predicament to the forefront of the medical community's consciousness.[61] It also led to physicians taking a more active role in patients' health by warning against the dangers of prolonged sitting.

Yet research in this area has been somewhat difficult due the limitation of self-reported sitting behavior and subjects' memory recall. A 2017 study was more definitive because it measured sedentary time with a hip-mounted accelerometer and studied nearly 8,000 Americans, ages 45 and older.[62] Similarly, this study found that (1) total amount of time spent being sedentary and (2) prolonged, continuous sedentariness was associated with increased risk of death. The one major difference was that getting up and/ or moving around every 30 minutes could potentially offset the bad effects of prolonged sitting. This has led us to the recommendation that people

---

61 Aviroop Biswas et al., "Sedentary time and its association with risk for disease incidence, mortality, and hospitalization in adults: a systematic review and meta-analysis," *Annals of Internal Medicine* 162, no.2 (January 20, 2015): 123-32.

62 Keith M. Diaz et al., "Patterns of Sedentary Behavior and Mortality in U.S. Middle-Aged and Older Adults: A National Cohort Study," *Annals of Internal Medicine* 167, no.7 (October 3, 2017): 465-475.

in desk jobs take regular breaks throughout the day. If you work eight to nine hours a day sitting in front of a computer, stand up, stretch, or walk around (or march in place) for a couple of minutes, at least once an hour (good), if not every half hour (even better). In case you were wondering, cigarette and e-cigarette breaks DO NOT COUNT.

ADDING MOVEMENT TO YOUR DAILY WORK ROUTINE

- Stand up while you talk on the phone.

- Use an adjustable standing desk that allows you to stand and then sit when you get tired.

- Use a specialized bike or treadmill-ready vertical desk or create a DIY version with a computer screen and keyboard above a treadmill or bicycle.

- When it's time for a bathroom break, take the long route.

- Take the stairs if you need to go between floors in your building.

- Do jumping jacks, squats, stationary lunges, pushups, dips, or run in place while you wait for your lunch to heat up in the microwave.

- Enlist co-workers for a quick 10- to 15-minute walk during your lunch break.

- Schedule two-minute stretch breaks during meetings—one break for every 30 minutes of meeting time—and put it on the agenda. If nothing else, it'll keep the meetings shorter.

Physical inactivity in general—not just too much sitting—is problematic and has far-reaching effects on the human body, including declining fitness and disease development.[63] And, whether by choice or by infirmary, being

63   Frank W. Booth et al., "Role of Inactivity in Chronic Diseases: Evolutionary Insight and Pathophysiological Mechanisms," *Physiological Reviews* 97, no.4 (October 1, 2017): 1351-1402.

inactive accelerates the loss of both cardiovascular fitness and muscle strength and lowers the age at which an individual develops his or her first chronic disease. When you're in this Stress State, your quality of life goes down, your healthspan is shortened, your mortality (death) risk is accelerated, and healthcare costs go up significantly. I'll expand on these in just a moment.

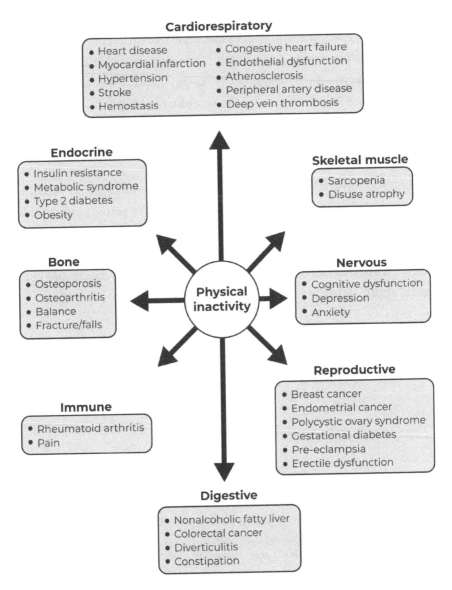

Too Much of a Good Thing?

The polar opposite to physical inactivity—over-exercising—can likewise be hazardous to your health, as it creates stress on the body. Aside from the obvious excessive wear and tear and risk of injury to the muscles, ligaments, and joints, over-exercising increases inflammation and depresses the immune system. Endurance athletes, such as marathoners and ultra-marathoners, are most susceptible to upper respiratory infections, arrhythmias, gastrointestinal bleeding, digestive problems, compromised kidney function, and sudden death.[64] Intense exercise can also lead to increased intestinal permeability ("leaky gut") and in extreme situations, it can cause heatstroke.[65] But for the rest of us, taking a day or two to rest every week is generally sufficient time to adequately recover and return the body to a state of homeostasis (i.e., reduced inflammation and normal immune functioning).

Common sense tells us that going from couch potato status to triathlete will not and should not happen overnight. If you're serious about adding more movement to your life, do it gradually and steadily, even if that means just walking at first. And if you are a true couch potato—especially an older one with a pre-existing condition—check with your physician and get his or her approval first.

*"If we could give every individual the right amount
of nourishment and exercise, not too little and not too much,
we would have found the safest way to health."*
—Hippocrates

---

64   Beat Knechtle et al., *Frontiers in Physiology* 9 (June 1, 2018): 634.

65   Glen Davison et al., "Zinc carnosine works with bovine colostrum in truncating heavy exercise-induced increase in gut permeability in healthy volunteers," *The American Journal of Clinical Nutrition* 104, no.2 (August 2016): 526-36.

Macro-Health Benefits of Movement

Achieving your Thrive State entails energy expenditure through movement. Whether you call it *physical activity* or *exercise* or *working out*, the physical and mental benefits can be tremendous when you incorporate it into your life. On a macro level, it's the big-ticket items like *quality of life*, *disease prevention*, *longevity*, and *anti-aging* which fall under the umbrella of "health and happiness" or "wellness."

As a physician, I am well aware that a significant portion of my patients do not exercise regularly despite my best efforts to convey the benefits. I am not alone in this regard, and U.S. government statistics seem to bear this out. The CDC's National Center for Health Statistics recently reported its findings from the 2018 National Health Interview Survey:[66] only 53.3% of Americans over the age of 18 met the Physical Activity Guidelines* for aerobic exercise (walking, cycling, jogging), and only 23.3% met the guidelines for both aerobic and muscle-strengthening exercise. As a nation, we have plenty of room for improvement.

Recommended Amount of Physical Activity for Adults

To attain the most health benefits from physical activity, adults need at least 150 to 300 minutes of moderate-intensity aerobic activity, like brisk walking or fast dancing, each week. Adults also need muscle-strengthening activity, like lifting weights or doing push-ups, at least two days each week.

SOURCE: Second Edition of the Physical Activity Guidelines for Americans, 2019

If 150 to 300 minutes a week sounds like a lot of time, it is really only a small fraction of the 10,080 minutes in a week. A commitment of 1.5 to 3 percent of your weekly time isn't so bad, is it? You're definitely worth it! But

---

66 "Early Release of Selected Estimates Based on Data From the 2018 National Health Interview Survey," National Center for Health Statistics, Centers for Disease Control and Prevention, www.cdc.gov.

if you need extra convincing, let's take a look at some of the macro-health benefits of movement.

General Quality of Life & Disease Prevention

General quality of life (GQOL) is an all-encompassing term that means different things to different people but from a research standpoint, entails the physical domain, psychological domain, social domain, and environmental domain. Research in this area tends to involve older adults because this is often when quality of life issues arise. A 2017 study demonstrated the positive impact of physical activity in a senior working-age (55-64) population.[67] The highest GQOL is associated with individuals who are most physically active, followed by those who are moderately active, and lowest in individuals who are the least physically active. With life expectancy in the United States hovering around 78.6 years, we should take these findings to heart.

Often, the physical domain in GQOL is the one which we have the most control over, and movement helps avoid the potential threats to good physical health and freedom. To clarify, I'm talking about this as freedom from sickness, disease, and disability. Regular physical activity during adulthood helps decrease the risk of suffering and pain from various conditions as we age. You may be predisposed to get a certain disease, but engaging in regular movement (and the other six BEEs) can potentially delay or prevent its development. If you already have a chronic or autoimmune disease, staying active can help manage it (decrease physical pain, reduce symptoms, halt disease progression).[68] Consistently meeting or exceeding the CDC's Physical Activity Guidelines leads to long-term health benefits.

---

67 Daniel Puciato, Zbigniew Borysiuk, and Michał Rozpara, "Quality of life and physical activity in an older working-age population," *Clinical Interventions in Aging,* 12 (October 4, 2017): 1627-1634.

68 Kassem Sharif et al., "Physical activity and autoimmune diseases: Get moving and manage the disease," *Autoimmunity Reviews* 17, no.1 (January 2018): 53-72.

Benefits of Regular Physical Activity		
Youth	Adults	Older Adults
General fitness Bone health Heart Health Improved cognition (ADHD) Reduced risk of depression	Reduced risk of death from all causes Reduced risk of heart disease, stroke, hypertension, type 2 diabetes & depression Bone health Improved physical functioning Brain health (decreased risk of dementia & Alzheimer's) Decreased cancer risk (bladder, breast, colon, endometrium, esophagus, kidney, lung & stomach) Decreased risk of post-partum depression	Reduced risk of falls Reduced risk of injuries from falls Decreased sarcopenia Improved cognition (dementia, Alzheimer's disease, Parkinson's disease)

"Movement is a medicine for creating change
in a person's physical, emotional, and mental states."
—Carol Welch

Longevity

Longevity refers to living a long life, or lifespan, but living longer doesn't always translate to living better, so I prefer to think in terms of healthspan. Here's what I mean: An individual's lifespan may be close to the U.S. average of 78.6 years, yet he or she may have spent the last five years in a state of poor health following a massive stroke. You could say this person's healthspan was only 73.6 years. Compare this with someone who was in a similar situation but whose stroke occurred 12 months prior to death;

this person's healthspan would be 77.6 years. No one would choose to live four extra years in poor health, especially if that meant extreme disability, suffering, and pain.

If we are to increase healthspan, our goals are not only to extend the period of good health but to compress the period of disease (morbidity) at the end of one's life. James Fries, Professor of Medicine, Emeritus at Stanford University, formulated the Compression of Morbidity hypothesis as a positive concept in the somewhat contradictory field of "healthy aging." His idea was clear—live a long healthy life with a relatively short period of decline just before death.[69]

Because regular physical activity helps stave off chronic disease and disability, it is an ideal strategy to achieve and remain in your Thrive State for as long as possible. Exercise, particularly strength training, helps prevent two conditions that occur naturally with aging—sarcopenia (loss of muscle mass) and dynapenia (loss of muscular strength). This alone is a tremendous benefit for the avoidance of acute injuries, such as falls, and shortening the recovery process after a fall or other skeletal injury (e.g., broken bones, back strain, or pulled muscle or ligament). Long periods of immobility following an injury can be difficult to bounce back from, so being in good physical condition before an injury will help prevent an acute injury from morphing into something more serious, such as fluid retention, pneumonia, weight gain, muscle atrophy, or depression.

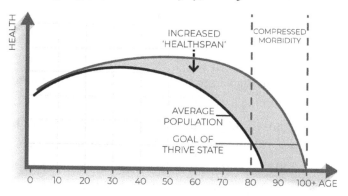

69   James F. Fries, "The theory and practice of active aging," *Current Gerontology and Geriatrics Research* 3 (2012) :420637.

Anti-Aging

When we're kids, we can't wait to get older and do all the things that adults can do, and when we, as adults, begin feeling the effects of aging, we wish we could do all the things we once did as children. Sound familiar? Probably no other time in history has our society been so focused on staying young and avoiding the deleterious effects of advancing age. So, while everyone's searching for the Fountain of Youth, why don't we look to our youth for answers? RUN. JUMP. SKIP. REACH. PLAY. MOVE. If we apply a slightly modified law of inertia—a body at rest stays at rest and a body in motion stays in motion—MOVEMENT is key to successful aging.

Exercise & Cognitive Anti-Aging

Maintaining cognitive function throughout life and especially in one's later years is a priority—period. Just ask anyone who's watched a parent, spouse, or good friend go through the ravages of Alzheimer's disease or other forms of dementia. It's heartbreaking to watch and terrifying to think that it may happen to us one day. Staying active may be our saving grace, although the research is not definitive at this time. However, a plethora of studies show that regular physical activity is associated with a lower risk for dementia and is also beneficial for people with mild cognitive decline.[70] Research provides valuable insight to assist practitioners to provide better exercise recommendations and encourage early action to increase cognitive healthspan. In some instances, "early action" means being active in youth and never stopping. Here are a few research highlights to ponder:

- Men with a lower level of cardiovascular fitness at age 18 had an increased risk of mild cognitive impairment and early-onset dementia later in life. If individuals had both low cardiovascular fitness and low cognitive performance at age 18, the risk was even greater.[71]

---

70   May A. Beydoun et al., "Epidemiologic studies of modifiable factors associated with cognition and dementia: systematic review and meta-analysis," *BMC Public Health* 14 (June 24, 2014): 643.

71   Jenny Nyberg et al., "Cardiovascular and cognitive fitness at age 18 and risk of early-onset dementia," *Brain* 137, no.5 (May 2014):1514-23.

- Women who self-reported as physically active at any point in their lives, but particularly as teenagers, were less likely to experience late-life cognitive impairment. If as teenagers, women were inactive but became active at a later point, their risk was lower than the women who never became physically active.[72]

- A 2016 literature search and analysis found that high physical activity (not moderate activity) had a protective effect on all types of dementia but more so for Alzheimer's disease.[73]

- Six months of supervised aerobic exercise (150 minutes per week) in patients with early stages of Alzheimer's disease yielded improvements in cardiorespiratory fitness, which were associated with improved memory and less atrophy in the hippocampus (the part of the brain involved with memory).[74]

- In 2018, the CDC reported that 11.2% of adults aged 45 and older and 10% of adults between the ages of 45 and 54 self-reported subjective cognitive decline (SCD), a condition that involves more frequent episodes and/or worsening memory loss or confusion. People aged 45 and older reported SCD at rates of at 13.8% and 15.2% for either living alone or having a chronic disease, respectively.[75]

Even if there is still disagreement in the research community about the effectiveness of physical activity on cognitive anti-aging, the knowledge that without a cure, 13.8 million Americans over the age of 65 will have dementia

72   Laura E. Middleton et al., "Physical activity over the life course and its association with cognitive performance and impairment in old age," *Journal of the American Geriatrics Society* 58, no.7 (July 2010): 1322-6.

73   Chris B. Guure et al., "Impact of Physical Activity on Cognitive Decline, Dementia, and Its Subtypes: Meta-Analysis of Prospective Studies," *BioMed Research International* 2017 (2017): 9016924.

74   Jill K. Morris et al., "Aerobic exercise for Alzheimer's disease: A randomized controlled pilot trial," *PLoS One* 12, no.2 (February 10, 2017): e0170547.

75   Christopher A. Taylor, Erin D. Bouldin, and Lisa C. McGuire, "Subjective Cognitive Decline Among Adults Aged ≥45 Years – United States, 2015-2016," Morbidity and Mortality Weekly Report (MMWR), Centers for Disease Control and Prevention, July 13, 2018, www.cdc.gov.

by 2050 should be a strong motivator to get moving.[76] In reality, cognitive anti-aging requires a multifactorial approach as does achieving your Thrive State. Lifestyle intervention consisting of regular physical activity and good nutrition, plus the management of cardiovascular risk factors, minimization of psychosocial stress, and treatment of major depression should be the focus for preventing dementia and cognitive decline.[77]

> *"The idea is to die young as late as possible."*
> —Ashley Montagu

Exercise & Aesthetic Anti-Aging

Body Composition

No one wants to be *old and fat*, so by remaining active throughout life, we can perhaps be *mature and good-looking*. It may just take a little more effort to maintain an appropriate body weight and muscle tone. Adequate sleep and good nutrition—which I've discussed in the previous two chapters—are still in play; although, your body may need slightly less sleep and fewer calories. Certainly, exercise is important to avoid sarcopenia and dynapenia, which contribute to muscle size, tone, flexibility, and ability to continue doing all things you did as a younger person. And don't forget the fat pounds that tend to replace the lost muscle pounds. This is why resistance training is so important for an overall exercise regimen and for aging muscles specifically.

Skin

Exercise makes the blood go round. The circulatory system plays a role in keeping you looking youthful by bringing nutrients and oxygen to the skin. Additional oxygen helps stimulate natural collagen production, which

---

76   "Facts and Figures," Alzheimer's and Dementia, Alzheimer's Association, alz.org.

77   Gopalkumar Rakesh et al., "Strategies for dementia prevention: latest evidence and implications," *Therapeutic Advances in Chronic Disease* 8, no. 8 – 9 (August 2017): 121-136.

plumps up the skin to minimize the appearance of wrinkles and fine lines. Exercise-induced sweating and increased lymph flow helps detox the body from poisons in food and in the environment.

Skeletal Integrity

Good posture, strong bones, and pain-free joints and back are all what I call "skeletal integrity." It's all the things that keep you vertically aligned, flexible, looking young, and having people scratching their heads about your age. Regular physical activity and minimal sedentariness—and the occasional chiropractor visit—are preventative maintenance for keeping your body in motion at any age.

Exercise for Stress Management

A great way to relieve stress is through any sort of physical activity that you find appealing—from light stretching, to yoga, to a leisurely walk, to something more intense. Regular activity reduces the body's stress hormones (cortisol, epinephrine) and increases the feel-good hormones (endorphins) for mind-body effects. Exercise can enhance your sense of well-being and at the same time, benefit your body by slowing heart rate, relaxing blood vessels, lowering blood pressure, and reducing muscular tension.

Micro-Health Benefits of Movement

Now it's time to get into the nitty-gritty science behind the health benefits of movement. Keep in mind that *it's the truth as we know it today*, and prevailing theories may change as we learn more.

From 1900 to 1940, at least two months of bed rest was the standard treatment for a heart attack; this was reduced to two weeks after research in the early 1950s showed that men put on bed rest following a heart attack were actually more likely to die than men who engaged in normal activity.[78] Nowadays, patients are out of bed the next day—if not earlier—and well on

---

78   S. A. Levine, "The myth of strict bed rest in the treatment of heart disease," *American Heart Journal* 42, no.3 (September 1951): 406-13.

their way to going home with a rehab plan in place. As we learn more about how the human body responds to exercise, the better we'll be at taking care of it, thereby remaining in the Thrive State with maximum healthspan.

Exercise & Insulin Resistance/Sensitivity

You've probably heard the terms *insulin resistance* and *insulin sensitivity* in relation to type 2 diabetes, prediabetes, and obesity but might be a little unsure which one is a good thing and which one is a bad thing relative to how they impact the body's ability to regulate blood glucose. The gist of it is: insulin resistance is undesirable; insulin sensitivity is desirable. As insulin resistance increases, blood glucose levels exceed the ideal range, and the risk of unhealthy metabolic conditions, such as type 2 diabetes, goes up. Conversely, as insulin sensitivity increases, blood glucose levels remain in the ideal range, and the risk of disease remains neutral or goes down.

Both insulin resistance and insulin sensitivity have to do with how the body utilizes insulin, so let's take a look at this important hormone. Insulin is secreted by the beta (β) cells in the pancreas after you eat a meal or snack containing carbohydrates. The carbohydrates are broken down in the G.I. tract, and one of the components is glucose, which moves across the bowel wall into the bloodstream. When the pancreas senses that there's glucose around, the β-cells crank out insulin to move the glucose into the cells where it can be used as fuel—either immediately by the muscles and for normal cell activity, or stored as fat for later use. Insulin is the "key" that opens the "lock" (receptor) to the "door" (cell membrane). In healthy individuals, this process is highly efficient, but with insulin resistance, not all the glucose gets into the cells. Some remains in the bloodstream, hence elevated blood glucose levels in people who either have diabetes or are on the way to developing it. Additionally, insulin levels in the blood are elevated since it is not being utilized.

Ongoing insulin resistance prompts the β-cells to secrete more and more insulin in an effort to decrease the amount of glucose circulating in the bloodstream. The β cells may become so overworked that their capacity for insulin production begins to diminish and some of them die off—that's an oversimplified explanation of what occurs with type 2 diabetes. The good news is that exercise decreases insulin resistance, increases insulin sensitivity, and decreases fasting insulin levels. And this is precisely why we prescribe regular exercise for people who are insulin resistant, have pre-diabetes, or are overweight.

Resistance exercise alone, resistance exercise plus aerobic exercise, and aerobic exercise alone have been shown equally effective in preventing adults with pre-diabetes from progressing to type 2 diabetes.[79] In patients who already have type 2 diabetes, aerobic exercise offers protective effects against diabetic complications and is viewed as a more ideal non-medical therapy since oral anti-diabetic medications are not without side effects.[80] Regular exercise is important to people of all ages, but it is critical in youth to limit the potential number of years or decades of insulin resistance and/ or full-blown type 2 diabetes. The more time that the body remains out of homeostasis, the more likelihood of diabetes complications. An analysis of 17 clinical trials showed that overweight children and adolescents may be able to prevent the eventual development of type 2 diabetes with exercise training, whether aerobic, resistance, or a combination; aerobic exercise was most effective, however.[81]

Exercise & Mitochondrial Health

Mitochondria are mini power plants within all living cells and generate the majority of the chemical energy—adenosine triphosphate (ATP)—used by cells to power the body's numerous functions. They also have domain over

---

79   Xia Dai et al., "Two-year-supervised resistance training prevented diabetes incidence in people with prediabetes: A randomised control trial," *Diabetes/Metabolism Research and Reviews*, (February 15, 2019): e3143.

80   Habib Yaribeygi, Alexandra Butler, and Amirhossein Sahebkar, "Aerobic exercise can modulate the underlying mechanisms involved in the development of diabetic complications," *Journal of Cellular Physiology* 238, no.8 (August 2019): 12508-12515.

81   Elisa Corrêa Marson et al., "Effects of aerobic, resistance, and combined exercise training on insulin resistance markers in overweight or obese children and adolescents: A systematic review and meta-analysis," *Preventative Medicine* 93 (December 2016): 211-218.

cell signaling, cell differentiation, cell growth, and cell death; they contain their own DNA and are self-replicating. In other words, they're pretty darned important, hence the name "cellular powerhouses." Mitochondria promote optimal cellular functioning, but if they are damaged, neurological disorders, muscle diseases, or endocrine diseases may develop. And as you may suspect, as you get older, the mitochondria's energy-generating capacity gradually decreases.

The good news is that exercise training may effectively halt aging at the cellular level by restoring mitochondrial health in skeletal muscle. A 2017 study examined high-intensity interval training (a 12-week biking regimen) and found that it could improve the age-related decline in skeletal muscle mitochondria by increasing the quantity of proteins that the mitochondria require to generate energy.[82] Study participants between the ages of 18 and 30 had a 49% increase in mitochondrial capacity, while those between the ages of 65 and 80 had a 69% increase; all ages had increased muscle size and improved insulin sensitivity. Because muscle cells accumulate a lot of wear and tear and don't readily divide, this research is promising. The hypothesis is that exercise will prevent mitochondrial deterioration in different types of cells and tissues, including heart and brain cells, which also wear out and are not easily replaced.

- Exercise stimulates the body's production of natural hormones and growth factors (growth hormone, IGF-1), which help maintain and build skeletal muscle.

- Exercise stimulates the brain's release of BDNF for improved cognitive functioning.

- Exercise prevents DNA degradation and prevents telomere shortening.

- Exercise helps optimize the gut microbiome for good G.I. health, brain functioning, and overall health.

---

82 Matthew M. Robinson et al., "Enhanced Protein Translation Underlies Improved Metabolic and Physical Adaptations to Different Exercise Training Modes in Young and Old Humans," *Cell Metabolism* 25, no.3 (March 7, 2017): 581-592.

Exercise, DNA, Epigenetics & Telomeres

Physical activity affects your genes—not the genes themselves, but the *expression* of those genes. Let's do a quick refresh on genetics/epigenetics before proceeding to the research. Your genome is your DNA that comprises your genes; it's what determines whether you have blue eyes or green eyes; brown hair or blonde hair. These traits remain fixed for a lifetime; in other words, if you were born with blue eyes, they don't change to green later in life. On the other hand, epigenetics ("on top of the genome") can alter how certain genes get expressed. Let's say you have a genetic predisposition—a "flag"—for obesity (your parents and siblings are all obese); if you eat poorly and never exercise, you'll likely wind up obese because the "fat flag" turned on the gene. But if, on the other hand, you eat healthy and exercise regularly, you'll remain an appropriate body weight because the "fat flag" did not turn on the gene. In this example, nutrition and exercise, or lack thereof, are considered epigenetic signals from your environment, and the good news is that these signals can be changed in a positive direction... by YOU and the lifestyle choices you make.

The research field of *exercise epigenetics* is quite young, and we are just beginning to scratch the surface when it comes to understanding how epigenetic signals alter the body's response to exercise.[83] One of the exercise-induced epigenetic changes in skeletal muscle is DNA methylation, a process in which methyl groups are added onto DNA molecules; DNA methylation plays a significant role in gene expression and helps establish the identity and function of cells as they develop and differentiate from one another. Of the many positive benefits of DNA methylation, its role in aging—or rather anti-aging—is that it represses aging and the development of cancer (carcinogenesis). As we age, the quantity of DNA methylation slowly decreases, so the goal of research is to explore whether regular exercise has a positive effect on DNA methylation. Stay tuned... This is sure to be the next hot topic in the science of exercise physiology.

---

83   Macsue Jacques et al., "Epigenetic changes in healthy human skeletal muscle following exercise–a systematic review," *Epigenetics* 14, no.7 (July 2019): 633-648.

Another related concept is that of the telomeres, or end-caps of your DNA strands, that gradually get shorter with age as cells divide over and over. You can think of telomeres like the plastic pieces at the end of shoelaces. While intact, the plastic keeps the shoelaces nice and neat, but if it falls off, the ends of the shoelaces become frayed. At some point, the shoelaces become too frayed that you throw them away and buy a new set. Intact telomeres stabilize the ends of the DNA and help prevent DNA degradation as the cells divide; the enzyme telomerase controls telomere stability and telomere length. Like the shoelaces, the telomeres may become so short that the cell no longer divides properly, and so the cell dies. Telomere length is generally used as a biomarker of aging—short telomeres indicate our cells are "old," and long telomeres indicate our cells are "young."

Longer telomeres are associated with healthy lifestyles, including exercise—and it's as simple as increasing the number of steps per day and reducing time spent being sedentary.[84] Longer telomere length, as measured in white blood cells (leukocytes) and skeletal muscle cells, is believed to be responsible for a lower risk of cancer, cardiovascular disease, chronic pain, diabetes, obesity, and stress.[85] Higher levels of physical activity have been correlated with longer telomeres. Studies with athletes show that they have longer telomeres than non-athlete counterparts. Exercise has a positive effect for anti-aging by maintaining telomere length and/or decreasing the speed and quantity of telomere shortening. A 2018 study merged two important concepts regarding telomere length and cancer: Shorter telomeres are associated with cancer, and having cancer is likely to increase sedentary behavior during treatment, which further contributes to telomere shortening.[86] It would not be unreasonable to extend this idea to other chronic diseases—an unhealthy, telomere-shortening lifestyle

---

84 Per Sjögren et al., "Stand up for health—avoiding sedentary behaviour might lengthen your telomeres: secondary outcomes from a physical activity RCT in older people," *British Journal of Sports Medicine* 48, no.19 (October 2014): 1407-9.

85 Nicole C. Arsenis et al., "Physical activity and telomere length: Impact of aging and potential mechanisms of action," *Oncotarget* 8, no.27 (July 4, 2017): 45008-45019.

86 Nikitas N. Nomikos et al., "Exercise, Telomeres, and Cancer: 'The Exercise-Telomere Hypothesis.'" *Frontiers in Physiology* 9 (December 18, 2018): 1798.

puts you at risk for XYZ disease, which, if you develop XYZ disease, causes you to become more sedentary and your telomeres to shorten more and at a quicker pace. This underscores the importance of remaining active throughout life. If you have a chronic or autoimmune disease, movement is even more critical.

Exercise & the Gut Microbiome

Do you recall in NUTRITION when we talked about how the gut microbiome functions better with a high microbial diversity and how eating a diverse diet helps provide that diversity? Well, it turns out that inhabitants of the microbiome also like it when you exercise. Physical activity is a non-pharmacologic intervention for increasing both microbial diversity and the sheer numbers of microorganisms, and this effect is independent of one's diet. Of course, that doesn't mean that your microbiome won't mind if you eat fast food and junk food as long as you exercise. You should be doing everything you can to remain in your Thrive State. Research shows that a lean person's microbiome is more responsive to aerobic exercise training than an overweight or obese person's microbiome; and longer duration or higher intensity exercise may be the key to optimizing the gut microbiome.[87] If exercise can positively alter the microbiome, it can improve the gut-brain axis, thereby improving mental health.[88]

The gut microbiome is still a relatively new field of study, yet it has enormous implications for patient health and the practice of medicine. In the non-so-distant future, physicians will likely practice the ultimate in concierge medicine—*personalized, microbiome-based lifestyle medicine*. Individuals will go

Dr. V's MOVEMENT Rx: Daily movement—whether light, moderate, or heavy intensity, structured or unstructured—has a wealth of physical and mental health benefits.

---

87 Lucy J. Mailing et al., "Exercise and the Gut Microbiome: A Review of the Evidence, Potential Mechanisms, and Implications for Human Health," *Exercise and Sport Sciences Reviews,* 47, no.2 (April 2019): 75-85.

88 Alyssa Dalton, Christine Mermier, and Micah Zuhl, "Exercise influence on the microbiome-gut-brain axis," *Gut Microbes* 10, no.5 (January 31, 2019): 1-14.

to their doctors for a baseline analysis of their gut microbiome, nutritional intake, and bloodwork, which will determine which exercise modalities and training regimens are best suited and most efficient for achieving the desired goals.

Pitfalls of the Weekend Warrior

Do you sit at a desk all week and then commit to a 100-mile bike ride with your younger co-workers on the weekend? It may have sounded like a good idea (or not a really bad idea) at the time, but waking up on Monday morning... well, you've decided otherwise. The good news is that you're waking up (you didn't expire). Exercise is associated with lower mortality, even for the weekend warrior who is active only one or two days per week.[89] This may come as a surprise to some, as local folklore dissuades sporadic vigorous exercise lest you have a fatal heart attack afterwards. A compelling study showed that one or two weekly sessions of moderate- or vigorous-intensity leisure/recreational activity was all that was necessary to reduce the risk of dying from cardiovascular disease (40%), cancer (18%), or something else (30%) compared with inactive individuals.[90]

Weekend warriors are, however, more at risk of injuries, including severe and fatal injuries, than individuals who exercise during the week.[91] This could result from (1) prolonged physically-demanding activity that exceeds one's exercise tolerance level, or (2) lower experience level with the activity. Generalized muscle soreness and lethargy may also be more common. A weekend warrior who experiences a debilitating injury (e.g., broken

Dr. V's EXERCISE Rx: Listen to your body when you exercise to avoid serious injury.

---

89   Eric J. Shiroma et al., "Physical Activity Patterns and Mortality: The Weekend Warrior and Activity Bouts," *Medicine & Science in Sports & Exercise* 51, no.1 (January 2019): 35-40.

90   Gary O'Donovan et al., "Association of 'Weekend Warrior' and Other Leisure Time Physical Activity Patterns With Risks for All-Cause, Cardiovascular Disease, and Cancer Mortality," *JAMA Internal Medicine* 177, no.3 (March 1, 2017): 335-342.

91   Derek J. Roberts et al., "The 'weekend warrior': fact or fiction for major trauma?" *Canadian Journal of Surgery* 57, no.3 (June 2014): E62-8.

leg, strained back) may inadvertently become sedentary for an extended period of time. If this describes you, take some common-sense precautions: Choose a few weekend activities to become skilled in doing; stretch and warm-up before starting; get a good night's sleep before and after; stay adequately hydrated; wear the appropriate protective gear; and know your limits. And, if possible, do some light exercise during the week—even if that means taking the stairs at work instead of the elevator.

What Type of Movement/Exercise Is Best?

The simplest (and honest) answer to this question is that the best exercise is the one that you'll actually do. It should really be something that you enjoy doing, particularly if the alternative is doing nothing. That being said, I'm going to review some forms of exercise that I've mentioned in this chapter or that were referenced in the studies I cited. Depending on your specific health goals and your current fitness level, select those activities that help move (pun intended) you towards your Thrive State.

Aerobic Exercise

Aerobic exercise is defined as sustained physical activity of low to high intensity that stimulates and strengthens the heart and lungs to improve the body's utilization of oxygen; this is why aerobic exercise is sometimes called "cardio." With aerobic exercise, you will breathe harder and faster; your heart will beat quicker than when you are resting; and you'll likely begin to perspire. Aerobic activities involve the large muscle groups, particularly the legs, and are rhythmic in nature. Examples include walking, jogging, medium- to long-distance running, swimming, and cycling.

For general health, moderate intensity exercise is recommended for 30 minutes three to five days a week; the 30 minutes can be broken down into three 10-minute sessions depending on ability level. Moderate intensity means that you should be able to easily carry on a conversation when exercising. Your heart rate and breathing will be quicker but not so fast that you have difficulty talking. For weight loss, continuous moderate to vigorous-intensity exercise for at least 45 minutes five to six days a week is recommended. Vigorous intensity means that your heart rate and breathing reach a level that you are only able to speak a few words at a time.

Resistance Training

Resistance training is defined as any exercise that involves muscles contracting against an external resistance or weight. These types of exercises increase muscle strength, tone, mass (size), and/or endurance (stamina). As a process, resistance exercises first break down or injure muscle cells (catabolism) and then repair, rebuild, and strengthen muscle cells (anabolism). The "external resistance" in resistance training can be rubber resistance bands, dumbbells, weighted bars, kettlebells, water bottles, cans of vegetables, or your own body weight. Resistance training is also referred to as weightlifting or weight training but does not always have the connotation of "bulking up."

Depending on your goals, resistance training can be utilized for muscle definition—a tighter, more sculpted, and physically fit appearance. To "bulk up," more resistance or greater weight can be used. By increasing muscle mass, you'll increase your metabolism and burn more calories at rest; assuming that you don't eat any extra calories, you will lose fat mass. Your body weight may stay the same or go up slightly due to the extra muscle mass, but you'll notice a difference in how much better your clothes fit you.

After age 30, otherwise healthy individuals begin losing muscle mass—as much as 3 – 5% per decade thereafter.[92] Many chronic diseases, including diabetes and obesity, are believed to accelerate the decline of both muscle mass and strength, thereby increasing the risk of sarcopenia and physical disability and decreasing healthspan.[93] For general health and to prevent sarcopenia in older adults, two days a week of resistance training is recommended. One day's workout should be devoted to upper body exercises and the other for lower body exercises.

---

92 "Preserve Your Muscle Mass," Harvard Health Publishing, February 2016, www.health.harvard.edu.

93 Rita Rastogi Kalyani, Mark Corriere, and Luigi Ferrucci, "Age-related and disease-related muscle loss: the effect of diabetes, obesity, and other diseases," *The Lancet Diabetes & Endocrinology* 2, no.10 (October 2014): 819-29.

High Intensity Interval Training (HIIT)

HIIT is somewhat of a new exercise strategy designed for maximal fitness compressed into a short workout. It involves alternating cardiovascular exercise performed with all-out effort/intensity followed by a brief recovery period of less intense exercise; this cycling between exercise and recovery lasts until the individual is too exhausted to continue. Workouts are typically less than 30 minutes, which benefits people with limited time. Exercises that work well with the HIIT model include a stationary bicycle, rowing machine, stair climbing, running, and uphill walking. A common HIIT regimen entails a 2:1 ratio of intense activity to moderate (recovery) activity. For example, 40 seconds of an all-out, maximal effort sprint alternated with 20 seconds of jogging or walking until exhaustion. Individuals of any cardiovascular fitness level can do a HIIT workout simply by modifying the activity and the time. A less fit person could alternate between 30 seconds of fast walking and 15 seconds of normal walking.

HIIT workouts improve athletic performance and as such, are beneficial for highly motivated professional and amateur athletes. Non-athletes experience significant health benefits as well, which are comparable or greater than those observed with moderate-intensity aerobic exercise. Studies of HIIT have demonstrated (1) improved glucose metabolism, especially in people with or at risk of developing type 2 diabetes, (2) decreased fat mass, (3) improved blood vessel function, and (4) improved cardiovascular fitness as measured by maximal oxygen uptake.[94,95,96,97] Because HIIT workouts

---

94   C. Jelleyman et al., "The effects of high-intensity interval training on glucose regulation and insulin resistance: a meta-analysis," *Obesity Reviews* 16, no.11 (November 2015): 942-61.

95   Stephen H. Boutcher, "High-Intensity Intermittent Exercise and Fat Loss," *International Journal of Obesity* 16, no.11 (2011): 868305.

96   Joyce S. Ramos et al., "The impact of high-intensity interval training versus moderate-intensity continuous training on vascular function: a systematic review and meta-analysis," *Sports Medicine* 45, no.5 (May 2015): 679-92.

97   Zoran Milanović, Goran Sporiš, and Matthew Weston, "Effectiveness of High-Intensity Interval Training (HIT) and Continuous Endurance Training for VO2max Improvements: A Systematic Review and Meta-Analysis of Controlled Trials," *Sports Medicine* 45, no.10 (October 2015): 1469-81.

can be intense, it's important to allow 24 hours between sessions to help the body adequately recover and avoid injury or overexertion.

Functional Movement

Functional movement is defined as the ability to move your body effortlessly and without pain. Proper muscle and joint functioning are key to biomechanically efficient movement that doesn't place any undue stress or create injury. Likewise, it's important to master functional movement before moving on to vigorous exercise so that the potential for injury is minimized. In functional movement training, several muscle groups are worked simultaneously to achieve better coordination and neuromuscular control. When the body functions as a stable, singular unit, it moves more efficiently and with regular practice, elicits a lean and toned physique. Functional movements include: deadlifts, front squats, kettlebell swings, lunges, planks, and squat presses. A great online resource to help you with functional movement is Functional Movement Systems (www.functionalmovement.com/exercises); the website offers videos of specific exercises and describes the purpose of each.

Flexibility

Joint flexibility describes the range of movement in a joint (e.g., elbow, knee) or a series of joints (e.g., fingers, toes), and the lengthening of muscles that cross the joint when a bending movement occurs (e.g., bending over at the hip). Flexibility is the reason a baby can put its foot in its mouth, and although flexibility decreases as most people age, regular stretching, yoga, and Pilates can help maintain or improve flexibility. The more flexible one is, the lower the risk of musculoskeletal injury and debilitating pain. Additionally, the effects of a sedentary or stressful workday can be helped by occasional stretch breaks.

Play / Spontaneous Fun

As children, we didn't think running around in the yard was anything but fun, but as adults we must give ourselves permission to play and have fun playing. That is... if we remember how to play. Think back to your own childhood or look to your children for guidance—a game of hopscotch, Twister, frisbee, basketball, or taking a turn on the jungle gym or merry-go-round. Play can be as light or strenuous as you make it and may burn a decent number of calories depending upon the duration.

> *"We don't stop playing because we grow old;*
> *we grow old because we stop playing."*
> —George Bernard Shaw

For Newbies: Getting Started on an Exercise Regimen

Although moderate physical activity (e.g., walking) is generally safe, I would be remiss as a physician if I did not give the standard advice to check with your doctor before beginning any new exercise program, especially if you have any of the conditions or symptoms listed. If it's been a while since you last participated in some form of exercise, begin with light activity, such as walking, and gradually ramp up your speed, duration, and frequency. If you're planning on vigorous activity, get the "all-clear" first. And if you're not particularly keen on exercise, refrain from calling it "exercise." Instead, call it "movement."

Check with Your Doctor Before You Begin an Exercise Regimen	
If You Have Diagnosed Diseases:	If You Have Cardiovascular Symptoms:
Heart disease	Pain or discomfort in the chest, neck, jaw, or arms at rest or with exertion
Type 1 or type 2 diabetes	
Kidney disease	Dizziness, lightheadedness, or fainting with exertion
Arthritis	Shortness of breath at rest, when lying down, or with mild exertion
High blood pressure	
Recently completed cancer treatment or are currently being treated for cancer	Ankle swelling, especially at night
	Lower leg pain while walking that goes away with rest
	A rapid or irregular heartbeat
	A heart murmur

Dr. V's Exercise Regimen for Thrive Status

I based my exercise regimen on science, not fads, so it's the truth as we know it today. Anyone can adapt my basic exercise regimen to fit their lifestyle and achieve their Thrive State. The key components are: (1) a weekly sprint at maximal effort; (2) resistance training with weights two days a week; (3) high-intensity interval training (HIIT) two days a week; and (4) low-level functional activity most days of the week. Here's how I put it all together:

Monday: Weights + low-level functional movement

Tuesday: HIIT + low-level functional movement

Wednesday: Recovery* + low-level functional movement

Thursday: Weights + low-level functional movement

Friday: HIIT + low-level functional movement

Saturday: Play

Sunday: A 20 – 30 second full effort sprint (repeat 5+ times) + recovery*

Be sure to allow 24 hours between HIIT sessions so the body can adequately recover. Vary your workout to suit your schedule and/or personal needs.

*Recovery activities include stretching, yoga, massage, or any light and relaxing activity that you enjoy.

Conclusion

"Exercise to stimulate, not to annihilate. The world wasn't formed in a day, and neither were we. Set small goals and build upon them."
—Lee Haney

No matter your reasons for exercising (e.g., reduce disease risk, manage a chronic condition, build strength, get fit, or look great naked), exercise, physical activity, and movement are vitally important to your Thrive State. Initially, I made the commitment to a new standard of physical exercise, in order to help myself overcome hypertension and type 2 diabetes. Mission accomplished. Now I'm fit, healthy, and like what I see in the mirror (naked, too!), and I look forward to an increased healthspan.

But I get it: it's easier to talk about exercising than to do it. Exercise is one of those BioEnergetic Elements, like sleep or perhaps even nutrition, where everyone intuitively understands the way forward. We all know we should be better at exercising—more consistent, more disciplined, more willful. But we don't always follow through. Instead, we sacrifice our commitment to exercise in order to make more time for other priorities: a night out with friends, a more relaxed morning with the children, or even just some well-deserved "you" time. And yet, we are only robbing from our long-term health and happiness—and meanwhile, pushing ourselves farther from the Thrive State and into a stressful state that impacts our cellular operations and even our genetic expression.

So, here is my proposal to you. I challenge you to make one change in MOVEMENT today; again, make it an easy one, even if it's for less than a minute if it will decrease your resistance to it. Even if you feel like there aren't enough hours in the day to get everything done, make time for yourself—and slowly build up to at least 30 minutes each day—to exercise. If you spend 8 to 10 hours a day creating wealth, spend at least half an hour creating health.

5 to Thrive

1. The BioEnergetic Element of movement and exercise is essential to the Thrive State. It optimizes your hormones as well as your cardiovascular and immune systems, promotes a healthy microbiome, improves brain function and detoxification, as well as prevents chronic disease.

2. Exercise is a powerful anti-aging medicine that promotes lean muscle, protects against injury, prevents cognitive disorders such as dementia, and supports telomere length.

3. If you work a sedentary job, take a break every 30 minutes to an hour to stand up and walk around.

4. Over-exercising can negatively impact your body and overall health. Taking a day or two of rest is typically sufficient for recovery.

5. Starting a new exercise routine, like a new eating style, starts with small, manageable changes. Make sure to integrate strength training and aerobic activity with a focus on flexibility and functional movements.

For additional resources on how to optimize movement and exercise, including fitness trackers and other biohacks, visit thrivestatebook.com/resources.

CHAPTER 7

MASTERING STRESS, HARNESSING YOUR EMOTIONS

You've undoubtedly felt stressed out at one time or another in your life, maybe even to the extreme of mental or physical *burnout*. If not, consider yourself extremely lucky, and read on so you'll know what the rest of us go through from time to time. Everyday demands, whether from school, work, career, family, or relationships, can create feelings of stress, or distress. Sometimes, stress can be acute or temporary, such as taking a test in school, interviewing for a new job, or spending the holidays with family. Once the situation is over, the unpleasant, stressful feelings go away. But when stress becomes chronic, such as working in a hostile environment, spending hours every day stuck in traffic, or dealing with an ill family member, stress can become harmful to your health.

STRESS AND EMOTIONAL MASTERY, the fifth BioEnergetic Element, is multifaceted and experienced differently across individuals; it is perhaps as individualized as individuals themselves. It is often the *perception* of stress that influences the degree to which we feel stress. Two people can experience the same situation yet have completely different perceptions of whether it was indeed, and to what degree, stressful. For example, two co-workers whose perfectionist boss routinely provides them equally with constructive criticism regarding their job performance: Co-worker A perceives it as criticism (distress), whereas Co-worker B perceives it as self-improvement advice (eustress). Perception has a lot to do with one's mindset, which I'll discuss in the next chapter, and perception also has quite a lot of influence on how we act—or react—to the stress. But for now, we'll focus on why stress is unhealthy—even life-threatening—and what you can do to get a better handle on it.

> *"Everyone has the ability to increase resilience to stress.*
> *It requires hard work and dedication, but over time,*
> *you can equip yourself to handle whatever life throws your way*
> *without adverse effects to your health. Training your brain*
> *to manage stress won't just affect the quality of your life,*
> *but perhaps even the length of it."*
> —Amy Morin

Effects of Stress on Health & Well-Being

Hormone Ping Pong

Common wisdom tells us that stress is bad for us, but do we really know *how* bad and *why*? Before I give you the scary statistics, let's begin by characterizing the body's physiological response when you encounter a stressful situation. You've probably heard of the fight-or-flight response, which was quite essential to human survival when our natural environment was far more physically dangerous than it is today. The sympathetic nervous system is responsible for rallying the troops and readying the body for the intense physical activity that soon follows.

A threatening situation (a stressor)—either one to fight against or to flee from—would trigger the hypothalamus to send nerve and hormonal messages to the adrenal glands to release voluminous quantities of adrenaline and cortisol (stress hormones). The sudden surge of adrenaline increases heart rate, blood pressure, respiration, and energy production so that we can take quick action to get ourselves out of danger. Cortisol increases the amount of circulating glucose in the bloodstream and in the brain; this helps fuel the muscles (for running away from predatory animals or fighting rivals trying to steal your food) and for quick thinking. Unnecessary body functions such as digestion, reproduction, and growth, are temporarily shut down, and immune system activity is suppressed.

Fortunately, the body's stress response naturally subsides once the threat is gone. Adrenaline and cortisol levels return to normal, and the body's functions resume a balanced, or homeostatic, state. Now, the parasympathetic nervous system takes over and stimulates the rest-and-digest, or feed-and-breed response. This complimentary response—a yin and yang, if you will—occurs at rest when danger no longer lurks. The body can go back to performing the now safe activities of digestion, urination, defecation, and sexual arousal, and the immune system gets back to work as well.

While we may not be fighting rival cavemen or running away from grizzly bears, modern-day stressors have simply evolved to remain relevant in our everyday lives. If these stressors are continually affecting us, the fight-or-flight response remains in high gear for long periods of time, which keeps adrenaline and cortisol levels chronically elevated. And that's where the health dangers come into play. Ongoing exposure to stress hormones disrupts the body's normal functioning and causes a loss of internal stability. Poorly managed or unaddressed stress can lead to an increased risk of mental issues (e.g., anxiety, depression, memory impairment, inability to concentrate), digestive problems (e.g., constipation, diarrhea), headaches, weight gain, sleep problems (e.g., insomnia), and heart disease. When those "unnecessary" body functions are shut down or disrupted for long periods of time, it's inevitable that health and well-being become compromised.

Stress Made Me Do It

Chronic stress can also lead to other unhealthy or risky behaviors. Many people eat mindlessly or eat fatty, high-sodium foods when they're stressed, which may lead to weight gain. Increased alcohol consumption can raise blood pressure and damage the arteries, lead to insomnia, or worse, cause dependence or vehicle accidents. Smoking harms the entire body and increases cancer risk. In other words, stress is bad itself, but also has great potential for harm in the behaviors it facilitates.

Behaviors Associated with Stress

- Agitated eating ("stress eating")
- Speaking more quickly than normal
- Racing thoughts & behavior but little accomplishment
- Excessive working
- Overextending oneself with little success
- Procrastination
- Sleep disturbances (too little or too much sleep)
- Physical inactivity
- Smoking
- Increased alcohol consumption

So, if you're not being chased by a grizzly bear, what is stressing you out? According to the American Psychological Association's (APA) 2017 statistics, the top five common sources of stress and percent of American adults experiencing them are: future of the nation (63%), money (62%), work (61%), political climate (57%), and violence/crime (51%).[98] Times have certainly changed. The 2017 APA stress survey was the first year to include *future of the nation* as a significant contributor to personal stress among Americans. Maybe being chased by a grizzly would be more enjoyable and, if nothing else, count towards your weekly sprint. Yet, in all seriousness, today's stressors are preventing people from reaching their Thrive States. If daily stress is keeping you in the Stress State, you must make changes, or the chronic stress will be as deadly as a grizzly bear—or a heart attack.

---

98 *Stress in America: The State of Our Nation*, American Psychological Association (November 1, 2017), Online PDF.

Stress & the Fire Within

Inflammation—the root cause of most chronic diseases—is the immune system's otherwise normal and helpful response gone awry. Nearly all chronic diseases are the result of too much inflammation in the body, but where exactly does all this inflammation come from? Inflammation is the purview of the immune system and at times, inflammation is very useful, like when you cut your finger or catch a gastrointestinal virus (i.e., food poisoning). The immune system initiates inflammation by creating pro-inflammatory cytokines (chemical messengers) in response to an injury or a foreign invader, a defense mechanism to protect you and get rid of the threat. This is all well and good—except when the inflammatory response continues well beyond resolution of the threat (e.g., your finger is healed, or you are no longer sick). It's almost as if the "inflammation switch" is permanently stuck in the "on" position.

Chronic inflammation contributes to autoimmune ("against self") diseases when the immune system mistakes normal healthy tissue for the foreign invader it's designed to protect you against. For example, in arthritis, the immune system thinks your joint tissue is under threat, so it responds with inflammation, and later antibodies, which over time damages your joints. In type 1 diabetes, the immune system attacks and destroys the insulin-producing beta cells in the pancreas. The immune system essentially turns rogue and goes against the body's own tissues, and for this reason individuals often have multiple autoimmune diseases simultaneously.

Psychological or emotional stress can also induce the immune system to produce pro-inflammatory cytokines. Research shows that acute stress stimulates production of interleukins—IL-6, IL-1β, IL-10—as well as tumor necrosis factor alpha (TNF-α).[99] The normal function of these cytokines is to attack viruses or bacteria, but if the "invader" is stress, then what is

---

99   Anna L. Marsland et al., "The effects of acute psychological stress on circulating and stimulated inflammatory markers: A systematic review and meta-analysis," *Brain, Behavior, and Immunity* 64 (August 2017): 208-219.

being attacked? That's a key question, as is: what happens when cytokine production remains chronically elevated (i.e., prolonged or chronic stress)?

The behavior of pro-inflammatory cytokines is to take care of the threat, whether it's a pathogen or acute psychological stress, and then disappear. So, with prolonged stress, these cytokines are circulating with more frequency and longer duration. This is believed to result in chronic, low-grade inflammation throughout the body, which in turn, leads to chronic disease and damage or destruction of various tissues within the human body. Of the diseases that cause the greatest morbidity (sickness and disability) and mortality (death), stress is ubiquitous in 75 – 90% of them.[100] The most common stress-related conditions affecting patients today include cardiovascular disease (e.g., atherosclerosis, hypertension); diseases of adverse metabolism (e.g., type 2 diabetes, non-alcoholic fatty liver disease); psychiatric and neurodegenerative diseases (e.g., depression, Alzheimer's, Parkinson's); and cancer.

Inflammatory bowel diseases, such as Crohn's disease, irritable bowel syndrome (IBS), and ulcerative colitis, have a stress connection as well; stress exacerbates these conditions by altering the normal secretion of digestive enzymes necessary for proper digestion and waste elimination. Additionally, corticotropin-releasing factor (CRF), a protein found in the brain and gut, was recently linked to stress as having significant influence over bowel function in IBS.[101] IBS research serves an important purpose since IBS prevalence in Western countries is quite high at 12 – 20% and greater than 20% in the United States.[102] At present, there are 58 prescription medications to treat IBS,[103] many of which you see advertised daily on television (Linzess, Viberzi, Zelnorm).

---

100 Yun-Zi Liu, Yun-Xia Wang, and Chun-Lei Jiang, "Inflammation: The Common Pathway of Stress-Related Diseases," *Frontiers in Human Neuroscience* 11 (June 20, 2017): 316.

101 Maria Giuliana Vannucchi and Stefano Evangelista, "Experimental Models of Irritable Bowel Syndrome and the Role of the Enteric Neurotransmission," *Journal of Clinical Medicine* 7, no.1 (January 3, 2018): E4.

102 Caroline Canavan, Joe West, and Timothy Card, "The epidemiology of irritable bowel syndrome," *Clinical Epidemiology* 6 (February 4, 2014): 71-80.

103 "Medications for Irritable Bowel Syndrome," Drugs.com.

In the same vein, there are 102 prescription medications to treat depression,[104] another condition that has ties to pro-inflammatory cytokines. Inflammation can lead to depression symptoms and/or worsen symptoms in people who are already depressed. Inflammatory markers can easily be measured in patients' blood, but mice studies show us what's happening in the brain. One particular study showed that exposing mice to stress triggered the immune cells in the brain, which led to rewiring of the neural circuits in the prefrontal cortex, and the mice developed depression-like symptoms.[105] Although we are not mice, our brains function in similar ways, and thus, this is another solid reason to avoid both inflammation and stress as much as possible. Statistics show that approximately 17.3 million American adults (7.1%) experienced at least one episode of major depression in 2017.[106] In life's big picture, depression will affect 15% of adults at some point in their lives.[107]

That formally brings us to the topic of *psychoimmunology*, the branch of medicine that studies the connections between the mind and the immune system. The very basic tenet of psychoimmunology—also called *psycho-neuroimmunology* (PNI) or *psychoimmunobiology*—is that mind and body are inseparable. Researchers in this field study the influence of emotions and the nervous system on immune function and how it relates to either onset or progression of autoimmune and chronic disease. As you can see, we've really been talking about psychoimmunology all along. When stress precipitates negative emotions (e.g., anger,

Dr. V's STRESS Rx: Chronic stress can lead to inflammation-related diseases. Take a proactive approach in addressing your stress head-on to ensure maximum healthspan.

104   "Medications for Depression," Drugs.com.

105   Eric S Wohleb et al., "Stress-Induced Neuronal Colony Stimulating Factor 1 Provokes Microglia-Mediated Neuronal Remodeling and Depressive-like Behavior," *Biological Psychiatry* 83, no.1 (January 1, 2018): 38-49.

106   "Major Depression," National Institute of Mental Health, U.S. Department of Health and Human Services, www.nimh.nih.gov.

107   Amy Morin, "How Many People Are Actually Affected by Depression Every Year?" Verywell Mind, March 19, 2020, www.verywellmind.com.

anxiety, fear, or sadness), the body undergoes physiological changes (e.g., heart rate, blood pressure) that affect other body systems. If stress is chronic, the body is unable to maintain its ideal state of equilibrium, and the immune system goes into overdrive and eventually, turns against the body it was designed to protect. Both quality of life and healthspan decrease.

Cells Get Stressed Out, Too

When you're dealing with chronic stress, it is not only your conscious mind that's having a bad day; your cells are too. You might be hurling swear words and profanities, but at the cellular level, there's a war among the neurons, microbiome, genes, and genes of the microbiome. The profanities are peptides, cytokines, and hormones. I already mentioned adrenaline and cortisol relative to the sympathetic nervous system response, but there are literally hundreds of chemical messengers involved in turning on the high-energy functions necessary for fight-or-flight. If these chemical messengers are being churned out continually, the affected cells suffer from imbalance. Remember, homeostasis is the preferred state of the human body. The body does a remarkable job of getting itself back to a homeostatic state, but sometimes the task is so overwhelming that catastrophic failure occurs—chronic diseases that may shorten healthspan and hasten death.

A Distressed Epigenome

Your genes may predispose you to a certain chronic disease, but through epigenetics, you exert influence over whether that disease is manifested or not. In other words, your actual genes have very little effect on chronic diseases. Chronic disease, in most cases, takes years or decades to develop, and your day-to-day habits and lifestyle—good or bad—push you towards disease or pull you away from it. It's not one cheeseburger a month that gives you heart disease; it's the daily cheeseburgers, plus the fries, and the 32 oz soda that give you heart disease. Likewise, it's not the one argument with your spouse that causes hypertension or depression; it's the daily arguing, verbal spats, denigration, and emotional stress that leads to chronic hypertension or depression.

Every chronic disease, including cancer and Alzheimer's, has its origins in a malfunction of the immune system. Too much inflammation or inappropriate inflammation is the result of an immune system that is not in its preferred homeostatic state. As a consequence, you are in a Stress State, as is your epigenome. Aging and psychosocial stress are associated with epigenetic changes and increased inflammation, and thus, increased chronic disease risk.[108] Because inflammation is probably the most influential determinant of whether a chronic disease manifests, the corrective course of action is to minimize inflammation in the body. Managing stress through one or more techniques on a regular basis throughout life helps keep the stress hormones and pro-inflammatory cytokines at bay.

If your life is controlled by stress—by choice or not—a good, err, *great* reason to get on top of it is for the sake of potential future offspring. Parental trauma and stress can cause epigenetic changes in children and grandchildren. Wow! That's scary. Research in this new field of *transgenerational epigenetics* isn't limited to just the negative epigenetic expressions, such as psychiatric disorders, but that is where science could have the most positive effect towards addressing offspring health and well-being.

Transgenerational epigenetics research has demonstrated trait transmission (e.g., depression, anxiety, PTSD) via both maternal and paternal lineage.[109] This has great significance for the offspring of military service members, migrants, victims of violence or abuse, and those suffering in poverty or undesirable socioeconomic situations. In the future, we are likely to see stress management as an integral part of a couple's preconception lifestyle, in addition to improved nutrition, weight loss, exercise, and detoxification. Mice studies have demonstrated early life stress fol-

---

108   Anthony S. Zannas et al, "Epigenetic upregulation of FKBP5 by aging and stress contributes to NF-κB-driven inflammation and cardiovascular risk," *Proceedings of the National Academy of Sciences of the United States of America* 116, no.23 (June 4, 2019): 11370-11379.

109   Shlomo Yeshurun and Anthony J. Hannan, "Transgenerational epigenetic influences of paternal environmental exposures on brain function and predisposition to psychiatric disorders," *Molecular Psychiatry* 24, no.4 (April 2019): 536-548.

lowed by exposure to enriching environments in male mice reversed the transgenerational epigenetic effect in their offspring.[110] This reaffirms the notion that our epigenome is not absolute and that positive epigenetic expression is within reach.

Stress-Induced Microbiome Alterations

Microbiome research remains in its infancy, but our fascination with the gut-brain axis is inspiring vast amounts of clinical study. Because we inherently realize the significant impact of mental stress in our daily lives, and we see how overwhelmingly debilitating it can be for some people, it makes sense that we would want to know more about how stress affects our gut bugs. Time spent in our mothers' wombs and early life is a critical developmental time for the nervous and immune system and is influenced by our mothers' gut bacteria. Much of this influence is transmitted during the vaginal birth process when newborns ingest and inhale mom's bacteria (in her vaginal secretions). Essentially, mom's bacteria seed our G.I. tract, so we hope she has bacterial diversity. It is the bacterial diversity and abundance that researchers are correlating with brain disorders and trying to understand how stress affects diversity and/or abundance of specific strains. This may eventually lead to better treatments, such as dietary approaches, supplementation, or fecal transplantation. (It's not as bad as it sounds!) Animal research suggests that introducing specific bacterial strains may actually reverse anxiety- and depression-like behaviors by balancing the neurotransmitters within the central nervous system and brain.[111]

Gut microbes from the species *Bacillus*, *Bifidobacterium*, *Clostridium*, *Escherichia*, *Lactobacillus*, *Lactococcus*, and *Saccharomyces* produce various neurotransmitters including acetylcholine, dopamine, gamma-aminobutyric

110   Katharina Gapp et al., "Potential of Environmental Enrichment to Prevent Transgenerational Effects of Paternal Trauma," *Neuropsychopharmacology* 41, no.11 (October 2016): 2749-58.

111   Ana Agusti et al., "Bifidobacterium pseudocatenulatum CECT 7765 Ameliorates Neuroendocrine Alterations Associated with an Exaggerated Stress Response and Anhedonia in Obese Mice," *Molecular Neurobiology* 55, vol.6 (June 2018): 5337-5352.

acid (GABA), norepinephrine, and serotonin.[112] Neurotransmitters are significant influencers of mental health, and alterations in the composition of the gut microbiome may be associated with neurological disorders, such as Alzheimer's disease, autism, depression, Parkinson's disease, and stress. Microbiome alterations have also been linked to changes in the transmission of neural signals in the hypothalamus and hippocampus, which contribute to the onset of anxiety and schizophrenia.[113] An imbalanced gut microbiome (dysbiosis) in early life has been hypothesized to cause increased susceptibility to stress-related disorders later in life, including PTSD following a traumatic event.[114] A 2017 exploratory study identified three bacterial strains—*Actinobacteria, Lentisphaerae,* and *Verrucomicrobia*—whose lack of abundance was associated with PTSD.[115]

In my discussion on nutrition, I noted that the gut microbes manufacture vitamins for use by the body, of which the B-vitamins are important to brain health and help remediate the negative mental effects of stress. Because the microbiome is such a significant source of B-vitamins, any alterations that decrease the microbiome's output of B-vitamins translates to an increased need for dietary intake, either through foods or supplements.[116] The human microbiome co-evolved along with us, and it synthesizes what the body and mind require for vitamin homeostasis. We should be mindful of how much the microbiome affects our health and care for it as we care for our other organs (e.g., heart, lungs, kidneys).

Lastly, an increase in cortisol secretion resulting from chronic stress can increase permeability of both the intestinal lining ("leaky gut") and the

---

112 Namhee Kim et al., "Mind-altering with the gut: Modulation of the gut-brain axis with probiotics," *Journal of Microbiology* 56, no.3 (March 2018): 172-182.

113 Xiuxia Yuan et al., "The gut microbiota promotes the pathogenesis of schizophrenia via multiple pathways," *Biochemical and Biophysical Research Communications* 512, no.2 (April 30, 2019:373-380.

114 Sophie Leclercq, Paul Forsythe, and John Bienenstock, "Posttraumatic Stress Disorder: Does the Gut Microbiome Hold the Key?" *The Canadian Journal of Psychiatry* 61, no.4 (April 2016): 204-13.

115 Sian M. J. Hemmings et al., "The Microbiome in Posttraumatic Stress Disorder and Trauma-Exposed Controls: An Exploratory Study," *Psychosomatic Medicine* 79, no.8 (October 2017): 936-946.

116 Stefanía Magnúsdóttir et al., "Systematic genome assessment of B-vitamin biosynthesis suggests co-operation among gut microbes," *Frontiers in Genetics* 6 (April 20, 2015): 148.

blood-brain barrier ("leaky brain"). This provides the pro-inflammatory cytokines more direct access to the central nervous system, and ultimately, the brain where they can inflame and damage neural tissue. Think of it this way: The castle is the brain. Cortisol lowers the drawbridge (tight-junctions) that is normally protected by a small force of guards (anti-inflammatory cytokines); the enemy (pro-inflammatory cytokines) can attack more surreptitiously when the castles defenses are down; and when cortisol secretion is chronic, the anti-inflammatory cytokines are overrun by the pro-inflammatory cytokines. Furthermore, if you have a gut infection or are taking antibiotics, which alter the microbiome composition, there may be more disruption between anti-inflammatory cytokines and pro-inflammatory cytokines and a more deleterious effect on the brain. The solution? Minimize cortisol secretion by lowering your stress levels. It's a good place to start, and I'll describe some strategies to help you get an upper hand on stress a little later.

Back on the topic of leaky gut and increased intestinal permeability... I can't stress enough the health dangers of this condition. We've only begun to scratch the surface in understanding how this pervasive condition is linked to autoimmune diseases. If you have any inflammatory-related condition, such as allergies, Alzheimer's disease, arthritis, asthma, cancer, Crohn's disease, diabetes, fibromyalgia, Hashimoto's, heart disease, irritable bowel syndrome, or Parkinson's disease, you more than likely have increased intestinal permeability. Even if you eat clean, avoid antibiotics, pain medications, and other gut-irritating pharmaceutical drugs, and avoid unhealthy habits, chronically elevated stress levels are still problematic. When the immune system is chronically activated (inflammation), your normally healthy tissues are targeted. It's been said that stress will kill you, but it's more likely that stress causes the inflammation that will kill you.

Emotional Control

You know the saying, "Shit happens"? Well, stress happens, too, and when it's particularly distressing, we need to establish emotional control. Unlike young children who have little to no control over their emotions, we adults do have control, or at least we should, in order to thrive. When some-one takes away a child's favorite toy, they cry (no emotional control). When someone rear-ends our prized sports car, we have emotional options that run the gamut—from yelling and swearing to calmly voicing our displeasure. Attaining emotional control gives us mastery over the instinctual emotional states and elevates us to the higher-functioning emotional states. By cultivating positive emotional states, we not only reduce our individual stress levels but the stress levels of those around us.

> **Dr. V's EMOTIONAL MASTERY Rx:**
> Keep an inventory of your emotions. List your negative emotions and positive emotions and their triggers. Have awareness on how to avoid your negative emotions, and do more of the activities that create the positive ones.

"The only thing you can really control
is how you react to the things out of your control."
—Bassam Tarazi

Emotional Control Disruptors (Negative Influences)	Emotional Control Enhancers (Positive Influences)
Poor lifestyle (sedentary, unhealthy eating, tobacco or drug use)	Healthy lifestyle (physical activity, good nutrition, not smoking, no drugs)
Toxic personal relationships	Respectful, nurturing personal relationships
Pessimistic attitude	Positive attitude
Unwillingness to expand one's horizons; mental stagnation	Desire to learn more; mental stimulation
Social isolation	Social interaction
Lack of education	Education and higher learning

Positive Emotional States

Making the case for cultivating positive emotional states is a no-brainer primarily because there's an abundance of evidence suggesting that negative emotional states are hazardous to your health; they contribute to the onset and/or exacerbation of chronic diseases by increasing production of pro-inflammatory cytokines.[117] Various studies have shown that negative emotions, such as hostility, rage, and anger, increase levels of IL-1β and IL-6.[118,119] Other studies correlate emotional states with immunity, and depending upon the context and duration of the emotion, there can be either beneficial or detrimental effects on a patient's health.[120]

If negative emotions contribute to immunosuppression, positive emotions, such as mirth and relaxation, are at least partially influential in immune protection by downregulating the production of stress hormones and pro-inflammatory cytokines. This has been observed in studies assessing the therapeutic benefits of laughter on mental health, particularly depression.[121] Laughter (mirth) decreases cortisol and epinephrine levels and increases dopamine and serotonin levels. In addition to self-reported stress reduction, improvements in natural killer (NK) cell activity has been observed in cancer patients.[122] Another study found that laughter upregulated 14 genes related to NK cell activity in patients with type 2 diabetes.[123]

---

117   Pietro Ghezzi et al., "Oxidative Stress and Inflammation Induced by Environmental and Psychological Stressors: A Biomarker Perspective," *Antioxidants & Redox Signaling* 28, no.9 (March 20, 2018) :852-872.

118   Mirko Pesce et al., "Emotions, immunity and sport: Winner and loser athlete's profile of fighting sport," *Brain, Behavior, and Immunity* 46 (May 2015): 261-9.

119   Jennifer Morozink Boylan et al., "Educational Status, Anger, and Inflammation in the MIDUS National Sample: Does Race Matter?" *Annals of Behavioral Medicine* 49, no.4 (August 2015): 570-8.

120   Samuel Brod et al., "'As above, so below' examining the interplay between emotion and the immune system," *Immunology* 143, no.3 (November 2014): 311-8.

121   JongEun Yim, "Therapeutic Benefits of Laughter in Mental Health: A Theoretical Review," *The Tohoku Journal of Experimental Medicine* 239, no.3 (July 2016): 243-9.

122   Mary P. Bennett et al., "The effect of mirthful laughter on stress and natural killer cell activity," *Alternative Therapies in Health and Medicine* 9, no.2 (March – April 2003): 38-45.

123   Takashi Hayashi et al., "Laughter up-regulates the genes related to NK cell activity in diabetes," *BioMed Research International* 28, no.6 (December 2007): 281-5.

A subsequent study by the same researchers found that laughter decreased post-meal blood glucose levels and blood levels of prorenin, a protein involved in the onset and/or deterioration of diabetic complications; it also normalized the expression of the prorenin receptor gene, something that is otherwise reduced in patients with type 2 diabetes.[124]

My own belief in the power of laughter led me to take on one of my favorite projects: launching and hosting Behind the White Coat, a comedic talk show that blends medicine, health, comedy, and Hollywood. In these videos—which are all available on YouTube (shameless plug)—I invite famous, not-so-famous, but altogether amazing people to share a stage and reveal their quirkiest human side through skits and banter on life, health, happiness, and whatever else blows our hair back. Laughter is truly the best medicine. As a doctor and a funny man, I finally get to prescribe it. In fact, that's my prescription for you: a daily regimen of laughter. You won't just be happier for it. You'll be healthier.

"Laughter is a bodily exercise, precious to health."
—Aristotle

Gratitude is another emotional state of great interest to medical professionals for its potential positive effect on health outcomes, although clinical data is relatively limited at this time. In one study of patients with asymptomatic heart failure, gratitude was shown to decrease inflammatory markers C-reactive protein (CRP), tumor necrosis factor-alpha (TNF-α), and IL-6.[125] Patients who expressed gratitude also slept better and experienced less fatigue and depressed mood. Another study measuring IL-6 levels found some evidence suggesting that gratitude attenuated some of the negative health effects in middle-aged American adults with low

---

124   Takashi Hayashi and Kazou Murakami, "The effects of laughter on post-prandial glucose levels and gene expression in type 2 diabetic patients," *Life Sciences* 85, no. 5 – 6 (July 31, 2009): 185-7.

125   Paul J. Mills PJ, "The Role of Gratitude in Spiritual Well-being in Asymptomatic Heart Failure Patients," *Spirituality in Clinical Practice* 2, no.1 (March 2015): 5-17.

socioeconomic status (SES) but not those with high SES.[126] Researchers hypothesized that by being grateful, individuals can buffer themselves against and mentally overcome life's daily stressors, particularly when SES makes them more vulnerable to certain diseases.

A close relative to gratitude, happiness has been correlated with IL-6 levels in adults with type 2 diabetes.[127] The happier patients had lower IL-6 measurements at baseline and after performing a mental stress test than their less happy peers. Further research is needed to determine whether a long-term state of happiness is protective for patients with diabetes or any other inflammatory-related disease.

> **Dr. V's STRESS Rx:**
> Your perception of stressful events or situations has a significant impact on whether you experience it as distress or eustress, so be mindful of what's going on in your life.

> *"Gratitude unlocks the fullness of life... It turns denial into acceptance, chaos into order, confusion into clarity... It turns problems into gifts, failures into success, and mistakes into important events. Gratitude makes sense of our past, brings peace for today and creates a vision for tomorrow."*
> —Melodie Beattie

Getting the Upper Hand on Stress

Before I share some successful coping mechanisms to help you get an upper hand on stress, I want to share which activities Americans, in general, are doing to deal with their daily stress. According to the APA's 2017 survey, "Stress in America™: The State of Our Nation," 14% reported smoking, yet thankfully, others are choosing more positive behaviors (www.stressin-america.org):

---

126   Andree Hartanto, Sean T.H. Lee, Jose C. Yong, "Dispositional Gratitude Moderates the Association between Socioeconomic Status and Interleukin-6," *Scientific Reports* 9, no.1 (January 2019): 802.

127   Laura Panagi et al., "Happiness and Inflammatory Responses to Acute Stress in People With Type 2 Diabetes," *Annals of Behavioral Medicine* 53, no.4 (March 20, 2019): 309-320.

- Listen to music: 47%
- Exercise or walk: 53%
- Pray: 29%
- Meditation or yoga: 12%

The APA survey indicates that many Americans acknowledge the importance of emotional support in coping with their personal stress, and 74% have a family member or friend to rely on for this support. Even though this percentage is high, 56% of those surveyed felt that they would have benefitted from additional support. The good news is that despite an increase in stress, more people are making a conscious choice to adopt stress-management strategies and gain greater emotional control.

Identify Your Stressors

A first step in stress management is identifying the stressors that are unique to you. Begin by identifying your stressors—the people, things, events, or situations that cause you to feel emotionally stressed—both in your home (or personal) and work (or school) environments. Make a list with two columns; write down the stressors you can change in one column and the stressors you cannot change in the other column. Eliminating the changeable stressors is easiest. Get rid of them—one at a time or all at once. As for the ones that you can't eliminate, commit yourself to a stress-management plan to better deal with those unchangeable stressors and act as the most authentic version of yourself.

General Practices for Minimizing Stress

- Avoid caffeine, alcohol, nicotine, and sugar.
- Get enough sleep (but not too much).
- Engage in physical activity, even if it's just to play.
- Try a stress-relief technique.
- Keep a stress journal.

- Find someone that you can really talk to.
- Practice time management.
- Don't over-commit yourself (just say no).
- Don't sweat the small stuff.

Stress Relief Techniques

Finding the stress relief technique(s) that works best for you may take some experimentation, and then mastery (lots of practice) of your chosen technique(s). It can be as simple as talking with a true friend, one who listens and who has sincere intentions towards your well-being. Or, in the absence of such a person, journaling—having that one-on-one conversation with yourself. If you don't enjoy writing, have that conversation in your head or out loud with yourself in a quiet, private space. (Doing it on public transport might not be such a good idea.) You may discover that multiple techniques are more effective or varying them from time to time is helpful. Stick with what works best for you, and don't forget about the setting.

People who spend time in nature (e.g., ecotherapy, forest bathing, green time, mindfulness in nature) just might be onto something profound when it comes to mental health. A growing body of research suggests that spending time in nature reduces stress and anxiety, improves mood, and increases one's sense of happiness and well-being.[128] Employees who commute through nature experience better mental health than those who don't, especially if they walk or cycle to get to work.[129] As modern societies become more urbanized, individuals have less opportunity for nature experiences; this is hypothesized to be a link between mental illness, particularly depression, and urbanization. A fascinating study examined neural activity in an area of the brain linked to mental illness risk and rumination

128   Margarita Triguero-Mas et al., "Natural outdoor environments and mental and physical health: relationships and mechanisms," *Environment International* 77 (April 2015): 35-41.

129   Wilma L. Zijlema et al., "Active commuting through natural environments is associated with better mental health: Results from the PHENOTYPE project," *Environment International* 121, pt. 1 (December 2018): 721-727.

(repetitive negative thoughts about oneself) in participants who either walked 90 minutes in a natural environment or walked 90 minutes in an urban environment.[130] The natural environment walkers had less high-risk mental illness neural activity and reported less rumination than the urban walkers. This suggests that *where* you practice stress management is just as important as actually engaging in stress-management practices to gain control over your life.

Exercise

Just about any type of exercise—from a casual walk to a maximal-effort sprint—helps relieve stress, and doing it in nature may increase the health benefit even further. Regular exercise/movement is a great equalizer against stress because it confers a protective effect against stress-related chronic diseases.[131] Exercise increases production of endorphins in the brain (the "feel good" neurotransmitters); decreases production of the stress hormone cortisol; helps relieve tension as you focus on the movement, rather than the stressor and negative feelings; provides renewed mental and physical energy; minimizes excessive inflammation; reduces symptoms of mild depression and anxiety; and improves sleep, which tends to suffer when you're in the Stress State.

Breathwork

When you're stressed, your breathing becomes quicker, and you take shorter breaths; this signals the brain to crank out more cortisol which, in turn, increases heart rate and blood pressure. Not good. So, returning your breathing to a homeostatic rate calms the brain, essentially telling it to stop releasing cortisol. Breathwork is the practice of consciously altering your breathing patterns (inhalation and exhalation) to reduce stress,

---

130 Gregory N. Bratman et al., "Nature experience reduces rumination and subgenual prefrontal cortex activation," *Proceedings of the National Academy of Sciences of the United States of America* 112, no.28 (July 14, 2015): 8567-72.

131 Marni N. Silverman and Patricia A. Deuster, "Biological mechanisms underlying the role of physical fitness in health and resilience," *Interface Focus* 4, no.5 (October 6, 2014): 20140040.

re-establish emotional control, and improve your mental state—all of which may translate into better physical health. Breathwork benefits people with psychiatric and stress-related medical conditions, including post-traumatic stress disorder (PTSD) and digestive issues.[132] There are various breathwork practices that utilize breathing exercises, such as pursed-lip breathing, diaphragmatic breathing or belly breathing, box breathing, 4-7-8 breathing, and alternate nostril breathing. Aside from stress reduction, these exercises help bring more oxygen to the body, thereby improving metabolism and facilitating toxin removal. Breathwork can be practiced anywhere at any time, even if you aren't stressed out.

Meditation

As a stress-management technique, meditation utilizes mindfulness (mental focus on a specific word, phrase, thought, activity, or object) to achieve an emotionally calm state. Meditation is often practiced in conjunction with deep breathing exercises and can be done sitting, standing, lying down, or while walking. Meditation has been practiced for thousands of years by various cultures and religions across the globe for self-awareness, enlightenment, and inner peace. Only more recently have Western cultures begun to recognize the health value of this Eastern tradition.

Pioneering integrative medicine practitioner Deepak Chopra, MD, is probably better-known as the personal transformation guru who introduced meditation to millions of people with his best-selling self-help books. His Chopra Center for Well-Being in Carlsbad, CA was the site for a 2014 study examining the effects of intensive meditation on mental health and epigenetic activity.[133] All participants were "on vacation" at the center, but only half received instruction and intensive practice in meditation. Everyone benefited from the "vacation effect"—suppression of stress responses and

---

132   Richard P. Brown, Patricia L. Gerbarg, and Fred Muench, "Breathing practices for treatment of psychiatric and stress-related medical conditions," *Psychiatric Clinics of North America* 36, no. 1 (March 2013): 121-40.

133   E. S. Epel et al., "Meditation and vacation effects have an impact on disease-associated molecular phenotypes," *Translational Psychiatry* 6, no.8 (August 2016): e880.

lowered inflammation, but the meditators' genes were expressed favorably with respect to cellular functions relevant to anti-aging and telomeres.

Meditation also has a positive effect on the gut microbiome, according to Dr. Chopra and colleagues at New York University and the University of California, San Diego.[134] The corticotropin-releasing hormone and catecholamine that are released when an individual is under psychological stress disrupts the gut microbiome, which under non-stress conditions produces short-chain fatty acids that have anti-inflammatory and anti-tumor activity. A non-homeostatic microbiome, in turn, negatively affects the neurotransmitters it is responsible for regulating; the gut barrier can also be compromised ("leaky gut"). Through meditation, chronic inflammation is reduced, and gut barrier integrity is restored. Because we are just learning how important the gut microbiome is to human health, meditation comes a close second to exercise in terms of prioritizing the numerous stress-management techniques available to us.

For many of us—including yours truly—meditation can be difficult because in daily life, we have been trained to be constantly on alert. As a doctor, I have been trained to scan for danger in every interaction. This means I'm always thinking and constantly fixated on danger. I know that many other professionals are mentally oriented the same way: from the lawyer whose career is built on constantly assessing liability, to the stock trader who is engrossed in up-to-the-minute fluctuations in the market. This is not a mindset that lends itself well to meditation!

For me, I found guided meditation to be a particularly useful entry point into the world of meditation. With guided meditation, someone is there guiding you through the process, directing you to pay attention to your breath and to focus in on certain aspects of your practice. With guided meditation, I felt like I had someone to help me transition into a regular practice, instead of jumping directly into the deep end myself. And today, through our computers or our smartphones, we can even practice guided

---

134 Ayman Mukerji Househam et al., "The Effects of Stress and Meditation on the Immune System, Human Microbiota, and Epigenetics," *Advances in Mind-Body Medicine* 31, no.4 (Fall 2017): 10-25.

meditation in our own homes. My personal recommendation for a place to start? The six-phase guided meditation process created by Vishen Lakhiani, the co-founder of MindValley.

Meditation can involve **creative visualization**, a cognitive process in which you conjure up positive mental imagery. This imagery may invoke feelings or emotions to help you address, resolve, or overcome physical, psychological, or social conflicts and limitations present in your life. Creative visualization could be described as using the power of your imagination to "heal" the unpleasantness—from physical injury and pain to psychological pain (e.g., sadness, depression, anxiety, fear)—and to "erase" the deficiencies—from low self-esteem to social awkwardness. Creative visualization allows you to access your subconscious mind and change those negative, unhealthy beliefs into positive, healthy beliefs. In this respect, it is similar to neuro-linguistic programming. This practice allows you to ultimately change your reality—to thrive.

I normally go through a morning routine that starts with five minutes of silence or creative visualization. To these five minutes, I often add an additional 15 – 20 minutes of guided meditation. Meditation is now a major part of my morning ritual to set my emotional state for the rest of the day. I think of it as my morning mindset routine. We have morning routines for many other aspects of ourselves—our morning dental routine, our morning skincare routine, or our morning health routine. We brush our teeth, put in our contact lenses, and perhaps fall to the floor for our morning push-ups. Why not approach our day's mindset with the same attitude?

Yoga

Originating in ancient India, the practice of yoga involves physical movements and poses that serve several functions, including strengthening the body; increasing flexibility; improving respiration, circulation, digestion, and hormone balance; clearing the mind; reducing stress; and strengthening one's emotional control. Unlike meditation with only a mental component, yoga has both a physical and mental component, and is thus sometimes considered exercise. Yoga—in its many forms—is often practiced in combination with specific breathing techniques and/or meditation. According to the APA survey, "Stress in America™: The State of Our Nation," 12% of people in 2017 used yoga or meditation to manage their stress, the highest percentage since the survey initially included it as an option in 2008.

A three-month study of participants at a yoga/meditation retreat revealed increased levels of brain derived neurotrophic factor (BDNF), a positive sign for brain health, as well as less self-reported anxiety and depression symptoms.[135] Another 12-week study of yoga/meditation found similar results in healthy individuals but with the added benefit of a reduction in the rate of cellular aging.[136] Reactive oxygen species (free radicals), cortisol, and pro-inflammatory IL-6 were reduced compared to baseline; total antioxidant capacity, BDNF, telomerase activity, and β-endorphin (brain protein with a morphine-like effect) were increased.

Tai Chi & Qigong

In Western culture, the lesser-known meditative movement practices of tai chi and qigong are utilized to enhance and balance one's "life energy," or qi (pronounced "chi"). These similar practices, of which there are many forms, are rooted in traditional Chinese medicine, philosophy, and martial arts and have been practiced for centuries for health-enhancement and fostering a calm state of mind. Much of the research suggests that Tai Chi and Qigong have positive effects on quality of life in healthy patients and those who are chronically ill.[137] The purposeful regulation of one's breath, mind, and body is believed to create a state which, in turn, activates an innate self-healing ability and stimulates the body's release of neurotransmitters.

---

135   B. Rael Cahn et al., "Yoga, Meditation and Mind-Body Health: Increased BDNF, Cortisol Awakening Response, and Altered Inflammatory Marker Expression after a 3-Month Yoga and Meditation Retreat," *Frontiers in Human Neuroscience* 11 (June 26, 2017): 315.

136   Madhuri Tolahunase, Rajesh Sagar, and Rima Dada, "Impact of Yoga and Meditation on Cellular Aging in Apparently Healthy Individuals: A Prospective, Open-Label Single-Arm Exploratory Study," *Oxidative Medicine and Cellular Longevity* 2017 (2017): 7928981.

137   Roger Jahnke et al., "A Comprehensive Review of Health Benefits of Qigong and Tai Chi," *American Journal of Health Promotion* 24, no.6 (July – August 2010): e1-e25.

Massage

Massage therapy involves the manipulation of soft tissues (i.e., muscles) as a way to relieve pain, muscular tension, anxiety, and depression symptoms. Psychological stress translates into tight muscles in the neck and back, hence the neck, back, and/or headache pain. Varying degrees of human or mechanical touch in a kneading-like fashion can assist in relaxation, causing one's stress to "melt away." In Western countries, the most common form of massage is Swedish or classical massage, although there are many techniques derived from Eastern cultures gaining in popularity (e.g., Shiatsu, Tuina). Sports massage is widely utilized by professional and elite athletes to reduce muscle spasms and fatigue and to expedite muscle recovery.

Research into the benefits of massage therapy remains somewhat conflicted, as some studies show positive effects and others do not.[138] A 2016 literature review found that massage elicits modest decreases in blood pressure in adult patients with hypertension and pre-hypertension.[139] Other research shows that this decrease is limited in duration to only a few days.[140] Nonetheless, massage therapy's calming effect is a non-pharmacologic alternative for a wide variety of patients—from preterm infants to children with behavioral issues to individuals in high-stress occupations to people

138 "Massage Therapy: What You Need To Know," National Center for Complementary and Integrative Health, U.S. Department of Health and Human Services, May 21, 2019, nccih.nih.gov.

139 I. Chen Liao et al., "Effects of Massage on Blood Pressure in Patients With Hypertension and Prehypertension: A Meta-analysis of Randomized Controlled Trials," *Journal of Cardiovascular Nursing* 31, no.1 (January – February 2016): 73-83.

140 Mashid Givi et al., "Long-term effect of massage therapy on blood pressure in prehypertensive women," *Journal of Education and Health Promotion* 7 (April 3, 2018): 54

with dementia.[141,142,143,144] Furthermore, as human beings, it's in our nature to enjoy loving, respectful physical contact.

Eye Movement Desensitization & Reprocessing

Eye Movement Desensitization and Reprocessing (EMDR) is a relatively new, sometimes controversial, type of non-talk psychotherapy used for treating patients with post-traumatic stress disorder (PTSD). American psychologist Francine Shapiro developed EMDR in the 1990s after making a chance observation that side-to-side eye movement seemed to reduce the disruption caused by negative thoughts and painful memories.[145] Although Dr. Shapiro recently passed away in June 2019, her work lives on through EMDR Institute Inc. (www.emdr.com) and the mental health professionals who work with former military combat veterans and victims of physical or sexual assault. Even those of us in the medical profession (e.g., emergency medical technicians and E.R. personnel) experience severe mental stress due to treating patient trauma and can benefit from EMDR.[146]

During EMDR therapy sessions, patients are directed to rapidly and rhythmically move their eyes side to side to tamp down the "power" of the memories of past trauma. EMDR therapy is endorsed by the Department of Veterans Affairs, Department of Defense, the American Psychiatric Association, and the World Health Organization. EMDR can also be helpful

141   María José Álvarez et al., "The effects of massage therapy in hospitalized preterm neonates: A systematic review," *International Journal of Nursing Studies* 69 (April 2017): 119-136.

142   Tiffany Field, "Pediatric Massage Therapy Research: A Narrative Review," *Children (Basel).* 6, no.6 (June 6, 2019) pii: E78.

143   Mahdi Mahdizadeh, Ali Ansari Jaberi, and Tayebeh Negahban Bonabi, "Massage Therapy in Management of Occupational Stress in Emergency Medical Services Staffs: a Randomized Controlled Trial," *International Journal of Therapeutic Massage & Bodywork* 12, no.1 (March 4, 2019): 16-22.

144   Felix Margenfeld, Carina Klocke, and Stefanie Joos, "Manual massage for persons living with dementia: A systematic review and meta-analysis," *International Journal of Nursing Studies* 96 (August 2019): 132-142.

145   EMDR Institute, Inc., *Eye Movement Desensitization and Reprocessing Therapy*, www.emdr.com/vita.

146   Mohammad Behnammoghadam et al., "Effect of eye movement desensitization and reprocessing (EMDR) on severity of stress in emergency medical technicians," *Psychology Research and Behavior Management* 12 (April 18, 2019): 289-296.

for patients, including children, who are too traumatized to talk about their stressful experiences.[147]

Psychotherapy

Traditional forms of psychotherapy (a.k.a. counseling or talk therapy), which require the assistance of a trained, certified, or licensed therapist, may be utilized for stress management if self-management techniques are not effective. Psychotherapy is not limited to people with a diagnosed mental illness; it can, in fact, help anyone who is experiencing distress caused by everyday life or major life events (e.g., divorce, death of a family member, job loss). Psychotherapists come in a wide variety, depending on their area of expertise, including psychiatrists, psychologists, licensed social workers, licensed marriage and family therapists, licensed professional counselors, and psychiatric nurses.

Finally... Take a Vacation

As if we didn't already know... vacations are good for your health, but now we have some scientific evidence. A 2019 study showed that taking vacations is good medicine because we experience them as positive events.[148] Specifically, vacation frequency played a role in reducing the risk of metabolic syndrome and symptoms (as measured by waist circumference, blood pressure, triglyceride and cholesterol levels, and fasting blood glucose levels). In fact, metabolic syndrome risk decreased by 24% in study participants who took an annual vacation, and for each additional vacation taken, there was an 8% decrease in the number of metabolic symptoms. I'd say that's pretty impressive and a good motivator to schedule a vacation, especially if you haven't taken one in a while. Fifty-two percent of American employees surveyed indicated that at the end of 2017, had unused vacation days;

---

147   Ana Moreno-Alcázar et al., "Efficacy of Eye Movement Desensitization and Reprocessing in Children and Adolescent with Post-traumatic Stress Disorder," *Frontiers in Psychology* 8 (October 10, 2017): 1750.

148   Bryce Hruska et al., "Vacation frequency is associated with metabolic syndrome and symptoms," *Journal of Health Psychology* 35, no.1 (June 2019): 1-15.

212 million vacation days were forfeited in 2017.[149] Make your earned and well-deserved vacation even better by including some other stress-reduction techniques—in nature, of course!

Dr. V's STRESS Rx: Practice stress-management techniques on a regular basis. When possible, do it in nature for optimal results.

Eustress

Do you remember earlier when I mentioned *eustress*? I wanted to end this chapter on a positive note: Not all stress is bad for us. Similar to how we think of "good" and "bad" cholesterol, the "good" stress is eustress. By definition, eustress is moderate psychological (e.g., a test) or physical (e.g., exercise) stress that the individual *perceives* as beneficial (not negative). The word was coined by Hungarian-Canadian endocrinologist Hans Selye, a mid-20th century pioneer in stress research.

When a stressful encounter or situation (the stressor) is viewed as a positive experience, it is perceived as a challenge rather than a threat. (Remember Co-worker B who perceived the boss' constructive criticism as being positive?) That is not to say said challenge is not uncomfortable or difficult, but it generally leads to personal growth and does not negatively affect one's health. Mindset is a significant indicator of whether the stressor is perceived as distress or eustress. If we are able to respond with a proactive attitude towards new challenges, seeing them instead as opportunities for growth, we can transform the stressors in our lives into bioenergetic positives!

Good news... the next chapter is devoted to mindset and how a change in thinking can benefit your own health and well-being. Mastering daily stress and transforming it into eustress is key to the Thrive State.]

---

149 "State of American Vacation 2018," U.S. Travel Association, May 8, 2018, www.ustravel.org.

Conclusion

"Adopting the right attitude
can convert a negative stress into a positive one."
—Hans Selye

Stress is a difficult enemy to combat. It arises at a moment's notice, our own minds produce it, and it is essentially invisible to the outside world. Equally invisible is the destructive effect of stress on our health. Chronic stress—that thing that we have all been taught to dismiss as an inevitable consequence of 21st-century life—has tangible negative effects on the body. Stress affects us on a microscopic level.

When we start to realize the consequences of these harmful effects, we start to understand that stress reduction is more than a quality-of-life issue. It is a health issue. (In fact, under the BioEnergetic Model, "quality-of-life" becomes essentially synonymous with our definition of "health.") This means that some of humanity's most time-tested treatments for stress, such as yoga, meditation, and Tai Chi, are actually health regimens passed down from some of the world's first healers!

If you take only one lesson away from this entire chapter, make it this one: there is no meaningful distinction between your long-term physical health, and your long-term mental and emotional health. If you are physically fit but chronically stressed, you are not healthy. I mean this as a statement of medical fact: your mental stressors will have physical consequences for your health and longevity.

That is why, under the BioEnergetic Model of health, lowering your own stress is mandatory, not optional. I encourage you to develop your own stress-management practice. You can start tonight, with your one change per chapter!

5 to Thrive

1. Stress and emotions have biochemical correlates that contribute to our BioEnergetic State and how our cells behave. Stress influences our hormonal systems and increases the levels of adrenaline and cortisol in our bodies, which can have disastrous health outcomes. Whereas positive emotional states activate hormones that promote a strong immune system and cellular healing.

2. Positively working on any of the other 6 BioEnergetic Elements has a synergistic effect in reducing our stress and improving our emotional states.

3. Stress can cause people to engage in unhealthy behaviors, such as smoking, overeating, and excessive alcohol consumption.

4. Parental stress can cause epigenetic changes in offspring—a great reason to reduce stress if you are planning on a family!

5. Stress reduction and emotional mastery can be acquired with non-clinical techniques such as meditation, breathwork, exercise, laughter, journaling, yoga, tai chi, qi gong, and vacationing. Psychotherapy and EDMR guided by professionals are also useful modalities.

For additional resources on stress and emotional mastery, visit thrive statebook.com/resources.

CHAPTER 8

MINDSET IS EVERYTHING

"Some people grumble that roses have thorns;
I am grateful that thorns have roses."
—Alphonse Karr

I finished writing the first edition of this book in early 2020, in the midst of the coronavirus pandemic. The virus is still a recent memory for all of us, but I suspect that we will each remember our experiences for a long time. For me, a certain moment stands out. It was March 16, and I had just returned from my shift at the hospital—our administrators were starting to implement new protocols, and I remember asking myself, *My God, what's next?* I was worried for my patients and what this dangerous new epidemic would mean for them. I had also heard the news that the stock market had taken a nosedive that day—nearly 3,000 points, a historic drop—and in the back of my mind I was starting to wonder what it meant for *me*, as well.

When I got home, I checked my computer—only to see that my investments for my retirement had taken a big hit. I found myself jumping between different tabs on my browser, and each one only brought bad news. New projections for the stock market, to breaking news about the virus, to updates from the hospital. With each click, I felt myself slipping deeper into a mindset of uncertainty and fear.

And like a lifeline to a man in quicksand, a certain quote—from the author Byron Katie—came to my mind. "Everything happens for you, not to you." So, I turned off my computer, sat down in a quiet space, and asked myself, *How is this happening for me? How can I turn this terrible situation into a gift?* The answer, I found, revolved around all the opportunities for digital connection that were already forming. In this time of physical isolation, people instinctively were reaching out for community. I could feel connected to people, perhaps even more connected than usual, even when I wasn't physically near them. This was, I recognized, something very special.

Then I went deeper, and I asked myself, *Why am I letting the number in my bank account—a number that I am simply staring at on a screen—have so much power over my emotional state?* I started to draw from some of what I had learned from my own personal journey to the Thrive State and from teachers like Tony Robbins and Vishen Lakiani. I asked myself: *What can I do right now, at this moment, to change how I feel? Is it calling a friend? Cooking a meal? Working out? What steps can I take, right now, to shift my focus?*

And, lo and behold, once I decided to shift my focus, to shift my *mindset*, I started to feel better. When I was focused on the fear and uncertainty of the situation, I felt paralyzed and demoralized. But when I focused on opportunity, gratitude, and joy, I felt more optimistic and energized. I was practicing the maxim that I preached: that *we* are our best medicine.

Our fifth BioEnergetic Element is MINDSET, the mental approach we take to our own lives. Life doesn't necessarily have to be as complicated as we tend to make it, especially if we can focus our attention on the positive aspects and adopt a more affirmative set of thoughts and beliefs. When it comes to health, how we *think* and how we *perceive* our health impacts how we deal with it. Has your current health state become your master, or are you the master of your health? Hopefully, by the end of this chapter you will feel more empowered to take control and make the changes necessary—the ones I've presented in the previous chapters—to lessen the effects of or prevent chronic disease and reach a state of abundant health, vitality, and optimal performance—the Thrive State. After all, YOU are your best medicine.

In Chapter 7: Mastering Stress, Harnessing Your Emotions, I introduced the idea that one's *perception* of a stressful situation or event is critical to dealing with it. Success or failure is determined by whether it's perceived as distress or eustress. Mindset is a broader concept which governs our overall reaction to all things—whether we find them distressing or not. If you think back to the two co-workers in Chapter 7, who both received constructive criticism from their supervisor, it is important to note that their individual mindsets played an influential role in how each perceived the specific event. Co-worker A had a limiting or fixed mindset, and her focus was on the criticism part (constructive criticism). Her mindset translated the experience into scrutiny and judgment. Conversely, Co-worker B had an open or growth mindset, and her focus was on the constructive part (constructive criticism). Her mindset translated the experience into genuine concern and motivation.

Now, take a moment and reflect on the last time you received constructive criticism. How did you deal with it? If it was with a limiting mindset, ask yourself: *Would I have done better with an open mindset?* If you answered "yes" (and I hope you did), you're one step closer to reaching your Thrive State. And by the way, you might want to ask yourself: *How was it intended?* It very well could have been offered with the most genuine of intentions.

Now, I'm going to share some of my personal experience with mindset to illustrate how I was "trapped" by the confines of my limited (fixed) thoughts and beliefs. My belief that I wasn't *enough*—enough successful, enough important—had me chasing money and significance, which only compounded the distress of trying to attain these attributes. Certainly, there's nothing wrong with desiring wealth or importance, but it was at the expense of my health. At the same time, I thought I was a fraud; no one would like the real me; and the world just wasn't being fair to me. Basically, I had the "woe is me" mindset long before I really understood what mindset really was. Our mindset and beliefs are the filter we use to give meaning and interpret our life circumstances, and it is the meaning we give to things that dictate our emotional states.

I now recognize that my early life circumstances—being a refugee from a poor family and whose parents didn't speak or act like everyone else—contributed to this negative mindset and influenced my self-defeating behaviors. It really wasn't until my health began to suffer significantly that I woke up to a sense of urgency. I needed to make a big life change. Yes, I needed to change my diet and exercise habits, but I also needed a mindset overhaul.

In order to get a handle on how to change my mindset for the better, I first needed to understand how mindset actually works. So, I narrowed it down to this: We all have a set of subconscious beliefs based on our early life experiences. These beliefs can be either empowering (positive) or disempowering (negative), and the external circumstances in our lives are filtered through these beliefs. What emerges on the other side of that filter is either eustress and positive emotions or distress and negative emotions. In turn, these emotions drive our behaviors—good or bad; healthy or unhealthy. When these behaviors become repetitive, they're referred to as habits, and because we're doing them over and over, they affect the epigenome and BioEnergetic State. In my case, I was getting a heaping serving of negative emotions, which not only has a direct effect on the epigenome but also led me to have additional bad health habits, which compounded the negative effects, leading to chronic disease. This is another example of how the bioenergetic elements can work synergistically to get you into either the Stress State or Thrive State; the outcome is ultimately all about the choices you make moment by moment by moment.

With introspection, I acknowledge that which I have always known... I had loving parents, and I realize that not everyone is as fortunate as I am. So, it would be a great disservice if I did not bring attention to the fact that many children are exposed to abuse, neglect, and household dysfunction that shapes their mindset. A major undertaking by the Centers for Disease Control and Prevention Kaiser Permanente's Health Appraisal Clinic in San Diego, CA in the late 2000s (The Adverse Childhood Experiences [ACE]

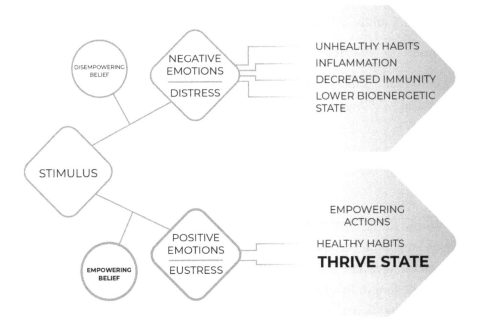

Study) demonstrated a link between violence-related stressors in childhood and risky health behaviors (e.g., alcohol abuse, illicit drug use, smoking, unsafe sexual activity) and adverse health outcomes in adulthood (e.g., alcoholism, liver disease, COPD, heart disease, sexually transmitted infections, depression, attempted suicide).[150] Subsequent research has demonstrated a link between ACE and poor mental and social well-being in adulthood, as well as lower life satisfaction.[151] Mindset has a significant impact on whether we feel satisfaction with life and to what degree.

---

150   Jennifer S. Middlebrooks and Natalie C. Audage, *The Effects of Childhood Stress on Health Across the Lifespan* (Atlanta, GA: Centers for Disease Control and Prevention, National Center for Injury Prevention and Control, 2008), Online PDF.

151   Elise Mosley-Johnson et al., "Assessing the relationship between adverse childhood experiences and life satisfaction, psychological well-being, and social well-being: United States Longitudinal Cohort 1995 – 2014," *Quality of Life Research* 28, no.4 (April 2019): 907-914.

Adverse Childhood Experiences (ACE)		
Abuse	Neglect	Household Dysfunction
Emotional	Emotional	Violence against mother
Physical	Physical	Household substance abuse
Sexual		Household mental illness
		Parental separation or divorce
		Incarcerated household member

Within the last five years or so, the idea of high ACE scores affecting telomere length has become an area of significant interest among researchers. Several studies have shown that ACE, particularly physical neglect, reduces telomere length in adulthood; other studies only observed this effect if the time frame between ACE occurrence and telomere testing was less than six years apart. Because ACE is relatively difficult to quantify, unlike telomere length, which can actually be measured, confounding results are not unusual. As research moves forward, there will undoubtedly be better methods developed to analyze the impact of ACE.[152, 153]

It is my sincere hope that whatever your current mindset is, it can be reprogrammed to be more open and towards growth, which will ultimately improve your health. Improving one's health is an ongoing *process of progress*. Try to resist feeling discouraged if it doesn't happen overnight—it most certainly won't. Think of the many years or decades you may have already spent living in a Stress State, so having an occasional lapse is OK. Getting to the Thrive State is a journey, an adventurous road trip with lots to see and do along the way.

---

152   Jason Lang et al., "Adverse childhood experiences, epigenetics and telomere length variation in childhood and beyond: a systematic review of the literature," *European Child & Adolescent Psychiatry* (April 9, 2019).

153   David Bürgin et al.,"Adverse Childhood Experiences and Telomere Length a Look Into the Heterogeneity of Findings—A Narrative Review," *Frontiers in Neuroscience* 13 (May 22, 2019): 490.

YOU are the Owner of Your Health (or "Unhealth")

The concept of YOU being the owner of your health is something you'll hear me return to over and over again. Even if you're not presently in the best of health, the good news is that you can definitely do something to change that, and your thoughts and mindset plays a big role. Bringing those subconscious beliefs to the conscious mind is key in figuring out why we do what we do. Once we migrate our thoughts and beliefs to a more open, flexible, and less judgmental mindset, then our external experiences produce positive emotions, positive behaviors, and positive habits, which recalibrate our epigenome to one that elicits good health.

Negative Beliefs Harm Your Health

You've probably heard that the mind can heal the body, but where's the evidence for this? Simple... it's called the "placebo effect," and doctors have known this for quite some time. In placebo-controlled clinical trials, one group receives the treatment (i.e., new drug) and the other receives the placebo (i.e., sugar pill). Participants receiving the placebo often report an improvement of their symptoms simply because they believe they had received the new "wonder drug." Placebo effects include measurable alterations in heart rate, blood pressure, and brain activity, as well as self-reported pain, fatigue, and anxiety.

The placebo effect is particularly strong in psychiatric disorders, including depression, anxiety, addiction, and even schizophrenia.[154] It has been noted that upwards of 80% of patients with mild to moderate depression reported an improvement of their symptoms when taking a placebo.[155]

Also, there's the "nocebo effect" when patients experience negative symptoms (e.g., headache, dizziness, nausea) in response to an inert sugar pill. This just goes to demonstrate the power of the human mind—an "if you

---

154   Ivan Požgain, Zrinka Požgain, and Dunja Degmečić, "Placebo and nocebo effect: a mini-review," *Psychiatria Danubina,* 26, no.2 (June 2014): 100-7.

155   Irving Kirsch et al., "The emperor's new drugs: An analysis of antidepressant medication data submitted to the U.S. Food and Drug Administration," *Prevention and Treatment* 5, no.1 (July 2002).

think it is, it is notion," so to speak. The placebo effect reinforces the power of positive thinking (i.e., hope and favorable expectations for future health) whereas the nocebo effect elicits physiological effects resulting from negative thinking (i.e., anxiety, fear, and negative expectations for future health).

Thus, we should take care when it comes to negative emotions and beliefs. Cardiovascular disease is highly correlated with negative emotions, which influence several areas of the brain that are involved with cognition, consciousness, and the experience of emotions.[156] Negative emotions trigger the fight-or-flight response and the release of cortisol and epinephrine. When the body is in a near-constant Stress State, its ability to self-repair is compromised and becomes more prone to infections and illness. So, negative beliefs and emotions could actually make you sick.

Mastering Your Mindset

Before I talk about ways to positively alter mindset, we should ask ourselves, *Can we indeed change our beliefs, emotions, and habits?* The answer is "yes," and the reason is because of a neurological phenomenon known as *neuroplasticity*, or *brain plasticity*. Neuroplasticity refers to the brain's ability to form new neurons and rewire neural circuitry in response to learning, or a new experience, or after a brain injury. Certainly, that's good news for anyone who has suffered a traumatic brain injury as a result of a stroke, car accident, or sports injury. But it's great (and very hopeful) news for individuals experiencing early-onset neurodegenerative decline or those who have neuropsychological disorders.[157] In the absence of disease, neuroplasticity offers a solution for individuals who truly want to own their health. Think of it this way: If we are what we eat, then we are also what we think.

---

156   Thomas E. Kraynak, Anna L. Marsland, and Peter J. Gianaros, "Neural Mechanisms Linking Emotion with Cardiovascular Disease," *Current Cardiology Reports* 20, no.12 (October 2018): 128.

157   Andrew Octavian Sasmita, Joshua Kuruvilla, Anna Pick Kiong Ling, "Harnessing neuroplasticity: modern approaches and clinical future," *International Journal of Neuroscience* 128, no.1 (November 2018): 1061-1077.

So, contrary to popular belief, your brain doesn't stop developing once you reach adulthood. It remains "plastic" throughout adulthood, although not as plastic as during infancy, childhood, and puberty. Imagine that your brain is made of soft plastic; it can easily bend in various directions without cracking or breaking apart. Now imagine that your brain is made of glass; it's nearly impossible to bend it without shattering it. The goal then, is to have a brain with plastic-like properties rather than glass-like properties, which, by the way, reminds me of the saying, "people in glass houses shouldn't throw stones..." Well, neither should people with glass brains.

Dr. V's MINDSET Rx: Changing your focus and the meaning you give to a particular situation will shift how you feel about it. Shifting how you feel will give you access to new actions you can take. Change your story, change your life.

The longer we can maintain neuroplasticity and positive mindset by opening the mind to new experiences and information, the better physical and mental health we'll enjoy. The emotions and habits that result from adapting to new stimuli (learning) will change old circuits and generate new circuits, as if upgrading the brain to a more sophisticated and efficient operating system. Here are some key beliefs that help elevate the human emotional states:

- *"The most important decision we make is whether we believe we live in a friendly or hostile universe."* —Albert Einstein

- *"Life is simple. Everything happens for you, not to you. Everything happens at exactly the right moment, neither too soon or too late."* —Byron Katie, author

- *"No matter what the situation, remind yourself 'I have a choice.'"* —Deepak Chopra, MD

- *"Live in the knowledge that you are a gift to the world."* —Debbie Ford, author

- *"Rename your 'To-Do' list to your 'Opportunities' list. Each day is a treasure chest filled with limitless opportunities; take joy in checking many off your list."* —Steve Maraboli, author

Professional Help vs. Self-Help

While I hope that this book will serve the "DIYers" well, everyone's emotional needs are different, and so I encourage you to do what works best for you. After all, you know you best. All I ask is that you be honest with yourself and commit to action, even if you're not quite sure whether it's the right choice. When faced with a fork in the road, the person who goes right instead of left can always turn around and take the other path—and pass right by the other person who still has not made a choice. Furthermore, a great deal can be learned along the detour—and be a source of knowledge to draw upon once the "correct" path is chosen. Now, let's get to the task of upgrading your mindset (or overhauling it, should that be the case).

The therapies and techniques I describe in the following pages are categorized into those that (1) require the assistance of a trained, certified, or licensed therapist and those that (2) can, for the most part, be practiced on your own or in a group setting (e.g., a public seminar). If you decide that professionally facilitated therapy is the right choice, be sure to research the practitioner's credentials and client satisfaction ratings. You can also request a referral from your primary care physician.

Avenues of Professionally Facilitated Personal Development

Hypnotherapy

In its simplest definition, hypnotherapy is the therapeutic use of hypnotism. Modern-day hypnotherapy has its origins in *mesmerism*, a technique developed by Austrian physician Franz Mesmer in the 1770s, who utilized it to treat patients with nervous disorders. In the mid-1800s, Scottish surgeon James Braid emerged as a pioneer in the field of hypnotism and hypnotherapy; today he is often regarded as the "Father of Modern Hypnotism." Today, hypnotherapy is considered a form of alternative medicine that, with the guidance of a competent practitioner, allows the patient to address a variety of issues, including stress management, breaking bad health habits, or resolving distressful issues from one's past. In general, hypnotherapy compliments other types of therapy for a well-rounded approach to mental and/or behavioral changes.

With respect to mindset and chronic disease, hypnotherapy can help a patient unearth and understand early life events that are manifesting within their current physical or mental health issues. For example, an obese patient undergoing hypnotherapy may discover that when he was a child, his family struggled with food insecurity and he was often hungry. Thus, his adult mindset was influenced by unconscious thoughts of fear, insecurity, and panic, which triggered his overeating, even though he was currently financially secure. Once the past issues are brought to the forefront, patients can begin moving forward towards a positive change of mindset. Mindset hypnotherapy—as it is often called—is not a one-stop solution and typically involves additional forms of psychotherapy and/or self-help techniques.

Eye Movement Desensitization & Reprocessing

As I detailed in Chapter 7, eye movement desensitization and reprocessing (EMDR) is typically utilized for patients who've had adverse childhood experiences or have been diagnosed with PTSD. By rapidly and rhythmically moving the eyes side to side, patients are able to tamp down the "power" of the memories of past trauma. Unlike hypnotherapy and other more invasive therapies, EMDR is useful for young children who are either too traumatized to talk about their experiences or are too young to adequately verbalize their trauma.

Controlled Substances & Plant-Derived Psychedelics

There is growing acceptance for the clinical use of controlled substances to treat mental illnesses. These include 3,4-methylenedioxymethamphetamine (MDMA, or Ecstasy) and medical marijuana for PTSD; Lysergic acid diethylamide (LSD) and psilocybin (mushrooms) for anxiety and depression; and ibogaine (iboga plant) for opiate addiction. Due to a high prevalence of PTSD today, MDMA has emerged as a favored treatment because it is gentler and more tolerable for the PTSD patient and enhances the patient's experience.[158] The shorter-acting MDMA helps the psychotherapist better manage the treatment session, and many patients are able to successfully access and process the emotional trauma with no neurocognitive side effects.

Although research has been limited to small sample sizes, MDMA-assisted psychotherapy holds great promise for patients whose PTSD has not responded to other treatments, including military veterans and first responders.[159] The Multidisciplinary Association for Psychedelic Studies (MAPS) (www.maps.org) was founded in 1986 by Rick Doblin to raise awareness and sponsor clinical research pertaining to the use of various psychedelics to treat PTSD and other mental disorders. The future direction of MDMA-assisted psychotherapy is projected to address substance abuse, and in particular people who use alcohol to self-medicate against childhood trauma.

Now, the stigma behind the use of these substances still exists today, though it seems like it is lessening every year. Which means you may be asking "Dr. V, have you had any personal experiences with psychedelics?" The answer is yes—and a positive one, at that!

Ayahuasca is a psychoactive tea brewed from the stalks of the *Banisteriopsis caapi* vine as well as the leaves of the *Psychotria viridis* bush. The psychoactive ingredient is Dimethyltryptamine (DMT), a molecule that our bodies naturally produce through the pineal gland but which can be found in other sources. Some people refer to DMT as the "spirit molecule," both because of its powerful psychoactive effects and because of how closely it links to religious or near-death experiences. When a person is dying, in fact, the body releases significant amounts of DMT—which is the medical explanation for why people who have been pulled back from the brink of

---

158   Ben Sessa, Laurie Higbed, and David Nutt, "A Review of 3,4-methylenedioxymethamphetamine (MDMA)-Assisted Psychotherapy," *Frontiers in Psychiatry* 10 (March 2019): 138.

159   Michael C. Mithoefer, "3,4-methylenedioxymethamphetamine (MDMA)-assisted psychotherapy for post-traumatic stress disorder in military veterans, firefighters, and police officers: a randomised, double-blind, dose-response, phase 2 clinical trial," *Lancet Psychiatry* 5, no.6 (June 2018): 486-497.

death report experiencing things like an altered sense of time or a feeling of supreme peace.

I tried ayahuasca three years ago. And before you ask, I tried it legally, thank you very much! (DMT is illegal in the United States. Obviously, you should know the law and obey the law with any controlled substance.) I was hoping for a spiritual experience of my own, to tell the truth. And the "spirit molecule" didn't disappoint. I experienced a powerful psychoactive effect from the ayahuasca: I felt that I could revisit experiences of my past, essentially reliving them with fresh eyes.

And I felt drawn to a certain experience in particular. Before I knew it, I was back on that boat, the one that took my parents and me out of Vietnam. Though I was only an infant and so would have only the haziest memories, I could suddenly remember everything with incredible clarity. I remembered what it had taken for us to escape, literally fleeing for our lives. I could see the fear and uncertainty etched on my parents' faces; I could sense all that it had taken for them to get there. I felt awash in love, compassion, and gratitude. All my old resentments towards my parents—the times they had discouraged me from pursuing my own paths; the pressures they put on me to succeed—washed away. I felt a new understanding for my parents—why they pushed me the way they did; the reasons for their decisions.

I have also tried Ketamine, the only currently legal psychedelic, and incorporated into my practice. Ketamine is a Schedule 3 prescription drug that has been safely used in anesthesia for decades. Many years ago, it was discovered that as anesthesia wore off, patients were having unique psychedelic effects. Ketamine is now being administered off-label by physicians for treating depression, PTSD, chronic pain syndrome, suicidal inclinations, as well as mental issues not considered clinical-level psychopathology. In my practice, those who have used Ketamine have reported enhanced mental performance, emotional mastery, and reconnection of purpose and self. Ketamine could enhance feelings of tranquility, openness, and radical acceptance, which can help individuals make peace with painful life circumstances and choices, whether historical or ongoing.

There are not a lot of medicines that can help someone forgive, heal past traumas, or repetitive negative thought loops. But the ones that can are powerful indeed. That is why I feel so encouraged by the increasing clinical use of some of these controlled substances for the treatment of mental illness or substance abuse. I believe that the future has more to offer when it comes to this type of treatment.

Avenues of DIY Personal Development

Here are some suggestions to help expand your mindset and change a narrowly focused belief system into one that is more encompassing, diverse, and potentially limitless.

The self-help world abounds with **self-help books, courses, seminars,** and **workshops.** There's a lot of quackery out there, but that doesn't mean that some of it isn't legit. What works for one person may not work for someone else, so I caution readers—go with an open mind and only proceed if your inner voice feels comfortable. Books are a great first step, and I recommend buying a highlighter (or two) to highlight the parts that resonate with you as you're reading through. You can always return to these key items for clarification, insight, or motivation.

One of my favorite online resources for personal growth and mindset reprogramming is Mindvalley (www.mindvalley.com). Mindvalley is a global school of more than 3 million people who benefit from personal development training courses aimed at increasing peak human performance in all aspects of life. Mindvalley founder and CEO Vishen Lakhiani is also a friend and mentor of mine, and I highly recommend his book *The Code of the Extraordinary Mind*. His mission is "to revolutionize the global education system by bringing new models of enhancing human potential to people everywhere and building a global school for Humanity 2.0."[160] Mindvalley is a monthly subscription-based service—think of it as Peloton® for your brain—and many courses are offered for free.

---

160   "Extraordinary By Design by Vishen Lakhiani," Mindvalley, www.mindvalley.com.

Vishen Lakhiani talks a lot about *culturescape*, or what he describes as "the web of beliefs, habits, practices, and mythologies of society that tell you how you should live your life." If you set goals based on your culturescape, you're, in fact, basing them on what society has programmed you to think you should be doing to achieve happiness instead of what will bring you true happiness. The solution is to redefine the way you set goals, and Vishen encourages people to ask three questions when choosing goals that will align with their happiness.[161] First: *What beautiful human experiences* do you want to have? Second: *What will help you grow* and become the man/woman you want to be? And third: *In what ways can you contribute* to others and the world as a whole? If you set goals with these three questions in mind, your goals serve your happiness—not your culturescape, and you will create an extraordinary life that's worth living every minute to the fullest.

Neuro-Linguistic Programming

Neuro-linguistic programming (NLP) derives from a branch of cognitive-behavioral psychology, and I place it in the category of *professionally facilitated self-help*. NLP was created by American motivational speakers and authors, Richard Bandler and John Grinder in the 1970s during the human potential movement. Bandler and Grinder hypothesized that certain linguistic, psychological, and behavioral qualities typify "great" people (vs. "not great" people), and that others could be trained to embody these qualities and become "great." In other words... duplicate what successful people do. The goals of NLP include improving one's interpersonal and communication skills in order to achieve personal and professional goals (e.g., peak personal development). Popularized by Tony Robbins in the 1990s, NLP's primary applications are in business, education, law, and medicine. Mind-training components focus on building self-esteem and confidence and eliminating fears and phobias. NLP's positive ideas have validity in themselves, but NLP techniques are also purported to be pseudoscience, or

---

161 Vishen Lakhiani, "An Alternate Model Of Goal Setting That Will Transform Your Life," Mind-valley Blog, May 28, 2019.

out of the mainstream practice of medicine, and various supporters have taken the original NLP concepts in divergent and competing directions.

With respect to health, NLP seeks to identify negative or limiting beliefs held by individuals who are in poor health. Patients are often directed to visualize themselves disease-free and in optimal health—as a more holistic way of enhancing the healing process. Neuro-Linguistic Psychotherapy (NLPt) utilizes NLP and specific interventions to treat psychological disorders and/or social problems and, according to researchers, is at least as effective as other psychotherapeutic modalities.[162] Books, audio tapes, and videos by NLP practitioners are available if you want to try self-treatment, but you should never rely upon these solely for treatment of a serious medical condition.

Neuro-Associative Conditioning

From the foundations of NLP, author and personal transformation expert Tony Robbins developed Neuro-Associative Conditioning (NAC), a system designed to change emotions and behaviors. The underlying premise is that human behavior is governed by (1) the need to avoid pain and/or (2) the desire to obtain pleasure. NAC involves creating a strong negative emotional state (e.g., emotional distress of having food poisoning) and pairing this overwhelming negativity with the desired behavior change (e.g., giving up sweets). Once this neuro-association is solidified, you clear it from your mind entirely, and then create a strong positive emotional state (e.g., emotional gratification of seeing a gorgeous sunset) without the behavior (e.g., no sweets). In other words, not eating sweets is now pleasurable; your new mindset has changed your new behavior. In full disclosure, Tony Robbins is not without controversy, both personal and legal, but his NAC model has helped many people achieve their goals, including the drivers of good health.

---

162 Cătălin Zaharia, Melita Reiner, and Peter Schütz, "Evidence-based Neuro Linguistic Psychotherapy: a meta-analysis," *Psychiatria Danubina* 27, no.4 (December 2015): 355-63.

PSYCH-K®

According to the originator of PSYCH-K®, Rob Williams, subconscious beliefs limit the expression of full human potential, such that your true identity is that of a spiritual being having a human experience.[163] Along with biologist Bruce Lipton, PhD, PSYCH-K® (www.psych-k.com) teaches that your beliefs and perceptions—positive or negative—affect your life at the cellular level, rather than your genes. Essentially, Dr. Lipton makes the case for epigenetics. PSYCH-K® is an interactive, non-invasive process to help change your self-limiting and self-sabotaging beliefs and elevate your consciousness to a higher state of functionality and creativity. Proponents claim that PSYCH-K® transcends the traditional practices of affirmations, positive thinking, and visualization to help facilitate positive behavioral change, induce stress reduction, increase sense of purpose and life satisfaction, and promote overall well-being for the benefit of the individual and of the world as a whole. PSYCH-K® originated in 1988 and draws upon some of the great intellectual and spiritual traditions from around the world.

Self-Service Experiential Options

"Once your mindset changes, everything on the outside will change along with it."
—Steve Maraboli

Traveling to other countries and experiencing different cultures is an excellent way to expose your mind to new ideas, thoughts, and beliefs. Even traveling from one state to another or from one coast to another can be quite an eye-opener among Americans. It's very likely to shatter the many preconceptions and stereotypes (false beliefs) we have about other people who are "different" from us. Such experiences not only change our mindsets but put us a step closer to wisdom.

Journaling can be a tool to allow your personal thoughts and beliefs to escape the confines of your mind and bring you clarity and self-awareness.

---

163   "Originator of PSYCH-K®," PSYCH-K International, psych-k.com.

Whether you put pen to paper or fingers to keyboard, journaling doubles as an effective problem-solving tool; use it to hash out conflicts between your own false beliefs and perceptions and to create solutions to match what really is. If journaling is a regular habit, go back and revisit past entries to see how your thinking has evolved over the months, years, or decades—you may be pleasantly surprised.

What I have found particularly helpful in the mindset mastery process is to have awareness of and **journal** my thoughts. If I find myself in a negative emotional state about a particular situation or circumstance, I get quiet and observe my thinking and the meaning I'm giving to that situation. Examples of some of my thoughts include: *I'm too old to start a new venture in life... Why do I always have all the bad luck... I'll never be as good as the greats on public speaking... I can't make money pursuing my passion... No one will really love me when they get to know the real me...* These thoughts are usually some form of "I'm not good enough" or "I don't belong." They are different for everybody.

Just journaling your thoughts gives you the power to have awareness that they are just thoughts—likely unconsciously adopted from the beliefs of the collective environment around you. With awareness then comes the power of choice and decisions to adopt more empowering beliefs which then lead to better emotions and inspired actions.

As I discussed in Chapter 7, **meditation** is an excellent stress-management technique that also promotes self-awareness and helps change mindset. Meditation helps clear any false beliefs, negative thoughts, or limiting thought patterns that are holding you back from true health. With the negativity gone, true beliefs, positive thoughts, and expanding thought patterns bring about new possibilities.

There are also **affirmations**, positive words or phrases you repeat to yourself as a personal mantra. Affirmations can help you to center positive emotions and behaviors in your own life. I am an affirmation-user (An affirmer? We may need a new term!) myself: most mornings, I repeat to myself that "I am grateful. I am playful. I am passionate. I am worthy." This affirmation is my own reminder of my self-worth, alongside my capacity for joy and gratitude. It has become a major part of my morning mindset ritual. The key here is to not only say them, but to feel the emotions associated with those statements as if they were true. Like when I say, "I AM Playful," I find myself feeling silly with a great big smile on my face, and likely doing a little silly dance. Does the Carlton dance ring a bell? (If you didn't get that reference, Google "Carlton dance and Fresh Prince of Bel Aire.")

Feel free to use my affirmations if you want, or find one that holds meaning for you... or make up your own! The most important aspect of an affirmation is that it resonates with you personally and you get yourself to feel it. Otherwise, your recitations will just be words without meaning. But if your affirmation works for you, that's all that matters.

Finally, never forget the power of **music** as a tool to alter your emotional state. After all, we all have that one song that puts us into a good mood. For me, anything with an up-tempo beat has a good chance of making me feel better. Music is an incredible tool not only for shifting your mindset, but for reminding you how easy it is to shift! We do not need sophisticated techniques, or gadgets, or cutting-edge science to put us in a better mood. We have the tools to do it ourselves.

So, queue up that favorite song... or if music doesn't work its magic on you, then maybe it's a particular smell or a specific

> **Dr. V's MINDSET Rx:**
> Changing your mindset to be more open, positive, and empowering is just as important as changing your diet to be more nutritious.

physical spot (like a park near your home) that brings you happiness. Use it! Think of it as your own cheat code for instant happiness. And believe or not, laughter, whether real or not, will activate endorphins and other neurotransmitters which will instantly make you feel better. In fact, Laughter Yoga is a practice involving prolonged voluntary laughter used as a modality to achieve positive physiological and psychological benefits.

In Buddhism, there is a concept called the "Bell of Mindfulness." When the bell is rung, the practitioner says to him/herself, "Listen! The sound of the bell brings me back to my true self." Within this practice is the reminder that it actually takes very little for us to remind ourselves that we should be happy. It's just a simple bell... or maybe in my case, a not-so-simple guitar solo playing in my earbuds. But these triggers do not make us happy. Instead, they simply unlock the happiness we already have within us—the happiness we must remind ourselves to feel. After all, your true self is a joyful self.

The Common Thread

There's no right or wrong technique to master your mindset. Whatever works for you *is* what works. As you go through life, you may pick up one technique, dabble in others, and at some point, you will find that one or two particular techniques are most effective at bringing about your own evolution. A common thread in all these techniques is (1) learning to release the emotional triggers that limit your mindset and perpetuate unhealthy behaviors; (2) removing the toxic relationships in your life (e.g., people, culture, religion); and (3) cultivating new thoughts, beliefs, and relationships that enhance your mindset so that you, in turn, can positively affect the people around you.

Forgiveness

It's been said that time heals all wounds, and while the passage of time may soften some people's emotional wounds, I'm more inclined to believe that actively removing your emotional triggers will encourage a more forgiving mindset. You're probably thinking to yourself right about now, Dr. V, that's easier said than done. Yes, I admit forgiveness is a pretty tall order, but in the long-term, you benefit—greatly. Acknowledge your negative feelings—they are real; they are your feelings; and someone did cause you harm—but don't allow your entire being to be consumed with negativity. By letting go of anger and resentment, forgiveness brings a sense of peace to your life and perhaps, even some compassion for the person(s) who hurt you. If that's not enough to convince you that forgiveness is a good option, there's research that shows forgiveness is good for your physical and mental health and helps counterbalance the negative effects of stress.[164,165]

Conversely, if you are the one inflicting the stress, don't underestimate the value of a sincere apology. Following an interpersonal transgression (e.g., verbal harassment), receiving an apology returns heart rate and blood pressure to pre-transgression levels more quickly than if you do not receive an apology; this effect is more significant in women than in men.[166]

It is easy enough for me to speak about forgiveness in the abstract. Yet I know that sometimes it can be very painful to find the courage either to ask forgiveness or to grant it to someone else. Yet unless we are literal saints—and I know I am not!—we will all do things that bring pain to others, at some point in our lives. Which means that we all carry the burdens of guilt, shame, disappointment, and regret.

These emotions do terrible things to not only our spirits but to our bodies on a physiological level. They have a massive effect on our bio-energetic state. Cortisol levels rise, immunities decrease, and inflammation increases. Forgiveness, then, is not just a spiritual practice but also a medical treatment.

One 'blueprint' for forgiveness that I have found inspiring is that of ho'oponopono, the indigenous Hawaiian prayer. Ho'oponopono is an ancient, ritualized practice, but at its core, ho'oponopono involves the repetition of these four phrases: "I am sorry. I love you. Please forgive me. Thank you". These four short sentences are the essence of any heartfelt apology. You can recite these words aloud to the person you have wronged, or—if you are unable or perhaps unready to say them in person—you can recite them in your heart.

---

164   Loren Toussaint et al., "Effects of lifetime stress exposure on mental and physical health in young adulthood: How stress degrades and forgiveness protects health," *Journal of Health Psychology* 21, no.6 (June 2016): 1004-14.

165   Kyler R. Rasmussen et al., "Meta-analytic connections between forgiveness and health: the moderating effects of forgiveness-related distinctions," *Journal of Health Psychology* 34, no.5 (May 2019): 515-534.

166   Matthew C. Whited, Amanda L. Wheat, and Kevin T. Larkin, "The influence of forgiveness and apology on cardiovascular reactivity and recovery in response to mental stress," *Journal of Behavioral Medicine* 33, no.4 (August 2010): 293-304.

I have witnessed acts of forgiveness that have helped people return to a state of greater emotional and spiritual peace. In turn, that peace creates the conditions for greater healing. I remember a powerful example from one of my patients: Todd (not his real name) was in his late 50s when I met him. He had a successful company and a legacy of professional success. He also had an aggressive case of liver cancer, with tumors appearing in new areas of the organ just as quickly as we could treat them. He was ineligible for a liver transplant because the cancer had already spread too quickly and too far—something that devastated our team when we found out. His chances of living the next five years, I estimated, were less than 10 percent.

It was soon after he learned that he was ineligible for a transplant that Todd began speaking to me of forgiveness. There were parts of his life that he had not yet resolved, he told me. He was estranged from his brothers, and he wanted to heal those relationships. It was impossible not to hear the unspoken end of these statements: *I must do this before I die.* I was there as Todd began composing a letter to each of his brothers, though at the time I was more concerned with reading his medical charts and the results of his newest round of tests.

But, sometime after, I noticed a change in Todd, a shift in his attitude and the way he approached things. At one point, we were discussing the results of his latest round of tests—tests which carried more bad news—and he told me that it was a strange thing. He felt he was nearing the end of his life, but that he had never been happier. His brothers were back at his side, and he felt at peace.

I was again reminded of Ishmael and the power we have to choose our own happiness. I was reminded of all the times I had seen my patients approach the end of their life with grace, dignity, and, yes, even joy.

But Todd did not die. My last treatment with him was over five years ago, and he has been tumor-free since then. He beat the odds. The less-than-10-percent odds, more specifically. As a doctor, I know that it would be premature to claim that his decision to forgive and to seek forgiveness from his brothers yielded tangible medical benefits. But I witnessed how a change in Todd's attitude presaged a change in his diagnosis, and I believe that Todd's newfound peace played a role in his recovery. Through forgiveness, Todd was able to change his BioEnergetic State, and his body was stronger for it, at a time in which he was battling for his life and needed every ounce of strength he could muster.

Create Space Between Stimulus and Response

I'm inspired to reshare the quote I presented in the introduction from Viktor Frankl: "Between stimulus and response, there's a space. In that space is our power to choose our response. In our response lies our growth and freedom." Our emotional responses are filtered through our subconscious programs—patterns of neural connections created from our past life experiences—to the stimulus of our life circumstances. If you are experiencing a negative emotional state, I have a process that may help guide a breakthrough. The first step is to take 10 long deep breaths; this will transform your physiology from that of a stressed state to a more parasympathetic state. This action will help you create space between stimulus and response. As you are breathing, have the awareness that your emotion is just a response of a learned pattern of neural connections. It is now in this space you've created with your breathing that you have the power of Choice. You can choose a new intention—perhaps an intention to take on a new empowering belief, an intention to change the meaning of a life circumstance, or an intention of how you want to feel or show up. And finally, from this new intention, take a new action. This action could be forgiving someone who has hurt you, choosing to be courageous and taking the action you fear (like public speaking), or performing an act of self-love. Actions taken consistently over time with intention will start to rewire new neural patterns, foster positive emotional responses, and

> **Dr. V's MINDSET Rx:** Taking new repetitive action towards a new empowering belief will rewire the brain toward this new belief. Neuroplasticity reassures us that we have the ability to heal the brain and the body through new thoughts, beliefs, and habits.

get you into the Thrive State. Remember, create space between stimulus and response, then ACT (1. Awareness, 2. Choice, 3. Take Action).

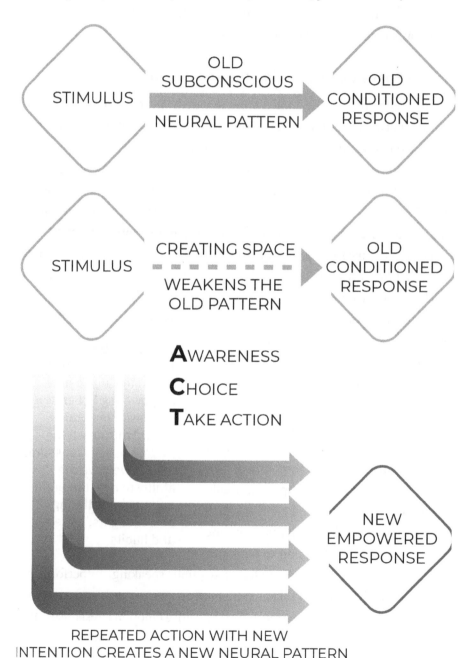

Conclusion

*"When you change the way you look at things,
the things you look at change."*
—Wanye Dyer

When we develop beliefs, emotions, and habits that allow us to thrive cognitively and emotionally, we improve our BioEnergetic energy and unlock the potential within ourselves to reach the Thrive State. To boil it down to its simplest distillation: happiness is healthy.

So, dedicate part of your individual health practice towards not merely countering stressful thoughts but to proactively developing a more positive and uplifting mindset. The health benefits will follow.

You can be forgiven for being a little daunted when I challenge you to make your one immediate change—per-chapter. After all, it's hard to implement a casual daily routine of forgiveness or gratitude. But tonight is the perfect time to try out a new affirmation or meditation (or an old piece of music!) It's also the perfect time to have a quiet check-in with yourself about what you have been carrying for too long. To guide you as you come up with your plan, I will list out a few BioEnergetic Enhancers and Detractors.

MINDSET ENHANCERS	MINDSET DETRACTORS
• An open mind, sense of curiosity, willingness to learn • Regular social engagement • Forgiveness • Upgrading belief systems • Awareness of subconscious beliefs that are affecting your emotions	• A closed mind with narrow focus • Resentment, anger • Indulging in negative thought loops • Remaining unconscious of disempowering beliefs

5 to Thrive

1. Mindset is the filter we use to give meaning to and interpret our life circumstances. This filter is built from our early life experiences but can be changed with continuous effort.

2. There are numerous avenues of personal development when it comes to changing our mindsets. Some of these are professionally facilitated, and some of these you can do on your own—like reading a self-help book, journaling, or taking an online course. The most important thing is to try different areas and see what works/what ideas speak to you.

3. When engaged in a negative neural thought pattern, create space between stimulus and response and ACT (1. Awareness, 2. Choice, 3. Take Action).

4. Forgiveness can bring us to a sense of peace in our hearts and minds, which can facilitate healing in the body. Ho'oponopono involves the repetition of these four phrases: "I am sorry. I love you. Please forgive me. Thank you."

5. Exciting advances in the field of psychedelic medicine are showing promise in a wide range of applications, including the treatment of mood, mental, and pain disorders as well as increasing brain neuroplasticity.

For additional resources on how to master your thoughts and mindset, including exclusive offers on some of the world's best programs, visit thrivestatebook.com/resources.

CHAPTER 9

ENHANCING THE RELATIONSHIPS
THAT ENHANCE YOU

Humans are naturally social beings, and relationships are what we do in life. Even before we emerge from our mother's wombs, we have a relationship with Mom. She provides us nutrition to grow and develop, and we (hopefully) provide her with an emotionally rewarding experience. After we're born, we rely completely on the care and interaction of parents, siblings, family members, and caregivers. We are simply the center of our own universes (and theirs)—something of a pint-sized narcissist. The relationships are one-sided, as we do all the *taking* and they do all the *giving*. As we grow up, the taking-giving ratio begins to change, our brain functioning matures, and we learn to initiate relationships on our own.

As the sixth BioEnergetic Element, RELATIONSHIPS and COMMUNITY are important to achieving our full potential—mentally, spiritually, and physically. Good relationships allow us to thrive, whereas bad ones can hinder and hurt us. When you feel good about your relationships, it's reflected in your health and vice versa. Most relationships begin on a positive note, even the ones that turn toxic. Initially, both parties are on their best behavior; no one wants a relationship to fail from the start. They hide their flaws and less desirable personality traits while trying to make a good impression. Unfortunately, when the good behavior phase ends, we sometimes find ourselves in non-productive and downright toxic relationships. On the other hand, positive relationships are ones that nourish both sides and help elevate us to a higher-functioning state... the Thrive State.

Let's explore the various types of relationships that contribute to our experience as social beings and that of belonging to a community of social beings. I'll also describe the health effects of such relationships so that you can chart a path forward.

Marriage vs. Singleness

Being married (or living as married), be it a heterosexual or same-sex relationship, can have its perks, as can remaining single. Whether you ask a married person, a single person, or both, you'll get lots of feedback on the pros and cons. There are innumerable influences on how and why the state of marriage and the state of singleness are recommended or not—previous relationship experiences; childhood experience with parents' marriage, divorce, or singleness; personal expectations; personalities; education; culture; religion, etc. All of this aside, the burning question is: Are married people healthier, and do they live longer than single people?

Conventional wisdom says, "yes," and medical sociologists tend to agree. Married men, and in particular, older married men benefit most; remaining married in adulthood protects them from premature death, and they're less likely to die from cardiovascular disease (CVD). One reason is that they do not experience elevated C-reactive protein (CRP) levels, an inflammatory marker and predictor of CVD.[167] Research shows that men typically fare worse when the relationship ends—either through death or divorce—than women. The belief is that when a relationship ends, stress levels go up, as does systemic inflammation. Women appear better equipped to deal with the stress, have more social support outside the marriage, and are less likely

---

167   David A. Sbarra, "Marriage Protects Men from Clinically Meaningful Elevations in C-reactive Protein: Results from the National Social Life, Health, and Aging Project (NSHAP)," *Psychosomatic Medicine* 71, no.8 (October 2009): 828-35.

to suffer from depression. On the other hand, men become more socially isolated, which often leads to risky behaviors such as excessive drinking, drug use, and unsafe sexual encounters.

Marriage also tends to benefit people who've undergone a health crisis, such as cancer, a heart attack, or heart bypass surgery. One study found that married men and women were two and a half times more likely to be living 15 years following their surgeries than unmarried men and women.[168] Furthermore, the couples who reported having a highly satisfying marriage were more likely to be alive than their unhappily married counterparts.

Health Benefits of Marriage or Long-Term Relationship (Cohabitation)

- More social support (less social isolation)
- More positive health habits
- Less risk-taking behavior
- Less alcohol and substance abuse
- High probability in the event of a health emergency that the other spouse can render aid or call for help
- High likelihood of having health insurance coverage

Non-marital cohabitation offers the benefits of companionship, which translates into similar health benefits.

A happy coupling may correlate with better health, but being married does not automatically guarantee happiness. Getting married for the sake of getting married doesn't benefit either party in the long run and may adversely affect the physical health status of both parties. This is particularly true for sexually transmitted infections (STIs). This may seem like a no-brainer, but research has confirmed that stable marriages protect men

---

168   Kathleen B. King and Harry T. Reis, "Marriage and long-term survival after coronary artery bypass grafting," *Health Psychology* 31, no.1 (January 2012): 55-62.

from oral and genital human papillomavirus (HPV) infections.[169] (I'm fairly certain the protection is bi-directional for the spouses of these men.)

Staying Healthy Together, Longer

- Encourage healthy habits – exercise or lose weight together
- Team up to break unhealthy habits – give up sweets or stop smoking together
- Pay attention – examine each other's skin for abnormal-looking moles or growths
- Schedule check-ups – go to each other's doctor appointments; take notes and ask questions
- Plan ahead – discuss end-of-life issues so that you can honor each other's wishes

Close Friendships

When it comes to close friendships and the Thrive State, two things are true: Good friends are good for your health, and quality is more important than quantity. So, if you only have a few dozen Facebook friends, don't despair, and don't feel jealous of the person with 500 friends either. True friends are the people who celebrate with you when things in your life are good and support you when things in your life are bad. More than just companions, they enhance your life and help you be a better person, and you reciprocate; true friendships are symbiotic.

Throughout life, close friends play an important role in each other's mental well-being and physical health. Major life events, such as divorce, serious illness, or death of a loved one are much easier to handle if you have a strong support system. In effect, a good friend is your best psychotherapist. Not only do friends provide emotional support; they encourage

169   K. M. Kero et al., "Stable marital relationship protects men from oral and genital HPV infections," *European Journal of Clinical Microbiology & Infectious Diseases* 33, no.7 (July 2014): 1211-21.

each other to take care of themselves by eating nutritiously, remaining active, avoiding alcohol and drugs—all of which help keep depression at bay. Friendships may be even more important as we get older and physical health issues arise. If a male spouse dies, single female friends may decide to share living arrangements to avoid loneliness, watch out for each other, and maintain a higher standard of living, knowing that they will likely live several more years.

If you do happen to have 500 Facebook friends, great! Maintaining connections with your online community can stimulate philosophical discussions and help relieve loneliness, but it may not translate to close offline relationships. Offline friendships have one significant advantage over online friendships, physical touch. And keep in mind the saying: "You can choose your friends but you can't choose your family." My advice: Choose wisely.

Strong Family Ties

Remaining close with family members is aspirational yet unrealistic for many people. In a perfect world, parents would get along with their children and siblings would get along with each other, but in reality, we have to make do with what is—or make changes. If your family relationships have you in the Stress State, make the necessary changes for you to thrive, even if that means putting some distance between or setting boundaries with relatives. It's certainly easier to dump toxic friendships than family relations, but for the sake of your mental health, do what's best for you. If you have children of your own, do your best to help them thrive at life. You can accomplish this by being a living example and incorporating the positive aspects of community into your own life.

Social Engagement (not Social Media Engagement)

Research shows that older American adults tend to live longer and healthier if they have a rich social life, and social engagement is important throughout life. A 2016 study analyzed data across four major studies with the aim of identifying any relationship between social relationships (e.g., social integration, social support, and social strain) and physical health biomarkers (e.g., blood pressure, waist circumference, body mass index, and C-reactive protein) within the framework of adolescence/young adulthood, mid-life, and late-adulthood.[170] The overall finding was that being more socially engaged or socially integrated in one's early and later life had a more pronounced positive effect on health. Early-life social connections could reduce hypertension and obesity in the later years. Researchers went so far as to say that social isolation has such a deleterious effect that it puts individuals at greater health risk than patients with type 2 diabetes.

This could be a function of our human experience. From birth through childhood, family is the center of our social universe; in adolescence, friends are the center of our social universe; in mid-life, career, spouse, and children are the center of our social universe; and in later life—for many people—friends re-emerge as the center of our social universe. Mid-life health may be more closely related to the perceived quality of one's social relationships rather than simply the number of social contacts. Once the busyness of mid-life (e.g., career, child-rearing, caring for aging parents) has passed, chronic disease creeps in during late adulthood. (Epidemiologists and some physicians argue that chronic

> **Dr. V's RELATIONSHIP Rx:**
> Seek out positive and rewarding relationships no matter where you are on the spectrum of life; your health will benefit greatly.

disease is a natural occurrence associated with aging, but I disagree. If you take this book to heart, you will age better with more vitality and sense of purpose.)

Loneliness in Older Adults

Actual and perceived loneliness and social isolation are associated with premature death, as well as being risk factors for physical and mental

---

170   Yang Claire Yang et al., "Social relationships and physiological determinants of longevity across the human life span," *Proceedings of the National Academy of Sciences of the United States of America* 113, no.3 (January 2016): 578-83.

illness in later life.[171,172] Circumstances which contribute to social isolation include illness, spousal death, family estrangement, impaired mobility, and declining financial resources. Studies utilizing the UCLA Loneliness Scale show that between 25 and 29 percent of community-dwelling (non-institutionalized) American adults over the age of 70 report that they are lonely at least some of the time.[173,174]

The high prevalence of loneliness in older adults suggests a need for intervention to improve adults' immunity to infection; to prevent, halt the progression of, or reverse chronic disease; to increase healthspan; and to prevent premature death. Motivating individuals to take care of their health through the various BioEnergetic Elements I've discussed thus far may be challenging unless social isolation is removed from the equation. And, by the way, this applies to younger people who find themselves socially isolated, perhaps only engaging online without the benefit of close friendships.

Social clubs (e.g., chess club, senior center, volunteer organizations) and special interest groups (e.g., gardening, computers, water aerobics) offered within the community are great ways to become a part of something and to overcome—or at least, set aside for a few hours—the feelings of loneliness and isolation. Face-to-face contact and conversation with people of similar interests does wonders for the mindset and helps relieve mental distress. Many of these activities involve mild physical activity, which helps maintain mobility and independence.

171   Julianne Holt-Lunstad et al., "Loneliness and social isolation as risk factors for mortality: a meta-analytic review," *Perspectives on Psychological Science* 10, no.2 (March 2015): 227-37.

172   Anthony D. Ong, Bert N Uchino, and Elaine Wethington, "Loneliness and Health in Older Adults: A Mini-Review and Synthesis," *Gerontology* 62, no.4 (2016): 443-9.

173   C. Wilson and B. Moulton, *Loneliness among Older Adults: A National Survey of Adults 45+*, Prepared by Knowledge Networks and Insight Policy Research (Washington, D.C.: AARP, 2010), Online PDF.

174   Carla M Perissinotto, Irena Stijacic Cenzer, and Kenneth E. Covinsky, "Loneliness in Older Persons: A predictor of functional decline and death," *Archives of Internal Medicine* 172, no.14 (July 23, 2012): 1078-83.

Pets

For many single people, animals provide a sense of relationship that facilitates their mental well-being. Pets are like automatic stress relievers and have proven effective in mediating symptoms of PTSD.[175] Dog owners get the added benefit of regular exercise—daily walks, lifting 50-pound bags of dog food, stretching to pick up poop, etc. Participating in all the responsibilities of owning a pet can provide purpose and structure, and while this is true for people of any age, it is especially important for older adults who feel lonely or have very limited social engagement. Taking one's dog to the dog park is an opportunity to meet and interact with other people who have at least one thing in common.

The Biology of Relationships

When you're in a good relationship, your body responds in physiological ways that enhance your overall physical and mental health. Conversely, toxic relationships slowly degrade your health and so insidiously that you may not even associate your physical symptoms with the state of emotional upheaval or abuse. Society, culture, or peers may imply that a bad relationship is better than no relationship, but if your body could talk—and it does—it would say otherwise.

Physical Touch

Physical touch is part of all healthy relationships—from a mother caressing her newborn, to a friend comforting a peer with a hug, to a caregiver holding the hand of a patient about to transition out of this life. Physical touch is how we communicate with each other, often without ever uttering a single word. In its many forms—caressing, massage, cuddling, hugging, kissing—physical touch benefits both the giver and the receiver when

---

175   Dessen Bergen-Cico et al., "Dog Ownership and Training Reduces Post-Traumatic Stress Symptoms and Increases Self-Compassion Among Veterans: Results of a Longitudinal Control Study," *The Journal of Alternative and Complementary Medicine* 24, no.12 (September 2018): 1166-1175.

offered with love and respect. With repetition over time, physical touch helps form a special bond between two people.

As a therapeutic modality, physical touch is being utilized for its positive effects on the immune system. In post-surgical patients, therapeutic touch significantly reduces pain and cortisol levels and increases natural killer cell activity, which improves immunity.[176] In patients undergoing cancer treatment, therapeutic touch helps prevent and/or treat the side effects of the anti-cancer treatment.[177] Massage therapy benefits for preterm infants in the NICU include improved brain development, increased gastric activity, better regulation of heart function, reduced risk of sepsis, shorter hospital stay, and less neonatal stress.[178]

When we're born, touch is the first sense we experience through acts of holding, snuggling, feeding, bathing, diapering, etc. As completely helpless beings, our ultimate dependency is connected to the touch provided by our parents and caregivers. Then as children, our independence begins to emerge, and our comfort level with physical contact and closeness begins to develop. We take cues from our family unit as we learn what is "normal" and what is culturally and socially acceptable touching.

By adulthood, we generally associate touching with connectivity and cooperation with others, and we are discerning in who we touch and how much based on the direct and indirect feedback we receive during such encounters. In other words, we are hopefully intuitive enough to gauge the other person's

> **Dr. V's RELATIONSHIP Rx:**
> Become proficient in the art of human touch.

"touchy-feely" level so as not to overstep. But if you do happen to err, offer an apology and try not to make the same mistake again. For most, though, the "human touch" is welcomed and conveys a sense of caring. When

---

176 Amanda Bulette Coakley and Mary E. Duffy, "The effect of therapeutic touch on postoperative patients," *Journal of Holistic Nursing* 28, no.3 (September 2010): 193-200.

177 Mathilde Gras et al., "Use of Complementary and Alternative Medicines among Cancer Patients: A Single-Center Study," *Oncology* 97, no.1 (2019): 18-25.

178 María José Álvarez et al., "The effects of massage therapy in hospitalized preterm neonates: A systematic review," *International Journal of Nursing Studies* 69 (April 2017): 119-136.

relationships turn romantic or intimate, more frequent and sustained touching enhances the experience for both parties.

Hormones

Marital satisfaction and stress affect the body's physiology. When researchers measured the daytime cortisol (a stress hormone) levels in married, never married, and previously married (divorced, separated, widowed) individuals they found some interesting results.[179] The currently married had lower cortisol levels overall, and cortisol rapidly declined in the afternoon hours. The hypothesis is that being relatively satisfied in a marriage accounts for less stress—hence, less cortisol secretion—than being in an unsatisfying marriage or not being married at all. The researchers' alternative hypothesis was that other factors led to lower stress levels, including more financial support, better access to healthcare, relative stability and routines, more positive health behaviors, and less risk-taking behaviors.

And speaking of hormones, the "cuddle hormone" oxytocin, which many people associate with maternal bonding, also enhances feelings of intimacy, affection, love, and trust in couples. Oxytocin acts as a neurotransmitter and secretion increases during intimate activities, especially in couples who are just beginning a relationship. Specifically, during orgasm, there is a rush of oxytocin for intimacy and bonding and a rush of dopamine for stimulating the reward center in the brain.

New research from Yale University has shown that a specific variant in the gene that controls oxytocin production affects the longevity of a marriage.[180] Interestingly, only one spouse needs this genetic variant for a marriage to be stable; both feel satisfied and more securely bonded to each other. Monogamy could then be considered a theoretical "side effect" of one or both spouses having this genetic variant.

---

179   Brian Chin et al., "Marital status as a predictor of diurnal salivary cortisol levels and slopes in a community sample of healthy adults," *Psychoneuroendocrinology* 78 (April 2017): 68-75.

180   Joan K. Monin et al., "Associations between spouses' oxytocin receptor gene polymorphism, attachment security, and marital satisfaction," *PLoS One* 14, no.2 (February 2019) :e0213083.

Oxytocin—much like serotonin and dopamine—exerts positive effects on mental health, particularly mood enhancement. In addition to promoting feelings of calm, contentment, and security (trust), oxytocin minimizes feelings of loneliness and sadness. These antidepressant-like and anti-anxiety-like effects may contribute to healthier marriages and coupled relationships in general—a possible explanation for the "no-drama" relationship.

Oxytocin isn't just for couples or mothers and their babies. Any type of positive human interaction stimulates the brain's production and release of oxytocin, and that's welcome news for everyone else who isn't coupled. Dave Asprey, author of *Game Changers* and founder and CEO of Bulletproof, suggests some simple modifications to our social engagement in order to get an oxytocin "fix." In order of oxytocin intensity, these are:[181]

1. Face-to-face communications
2. Videoconferencing
3. Talking on the phone
4. Texting
5. Posting on social media

Additionally, Dave Asprey's recommendation of more hugging and less handshaking is predicated on oxytocin release; however, my inclination is to ask permission first, especially if you are meeting someone for the first time. Cultural, religious, and familial norms often dictate how much personal contact is acceptable, so rather than risk offending someone, be respectful and pay attention to subtle cues. A smile and "May I offer you a hug?" usually get you the go-ahead signal, but if it doesn't, that's OK. Maybe your next encounter will, particularly if the other person gets to know you better and comes to view you as authentic.

But perhaps you have the opposite problem—hugging doesn't come naturally to you, or perhaps it is not part of your dynamic with your loved ones. I can relate because, as I mentioned earlier in this book, I did not grow

---

181   Dave Asprey, *Game Changers* (New York: HarperCollins Publishers, 2018).

up in a family where hugging was in major supply. So, the most personal piece of advice I can give about hugging is this: if you want to hug or be hugged by someone you love, don't be afraid to let them know.

Let's Talk About Sex

I have some great news for you: sex is good for your BioEnergetic State. (If you were weighing the medical benefits of a vow of celibacy, this announcement may be particularly welcome!)

As we just discussed, one of the main medical benefits of sex is its role as a major oxytocin booster. Yet this is just one of many benefits linked to sex. Sex is good cardiac exercise, is linked to a decreased risk of heart disease, lowers blood pressure, reduces the risk of certain cancers, and has even been found to help prevent colds and flu by promoting antibody production. There's a large body of research detailing both the physical and emotional benefits of sex; thus, you should consider your libido an important part of your overall health.

In my practice, I have a lot of clients who come to me with low libido or sexual dysfunction. The reasons for their low libido can vary wildly; it could be poor physical health, or an all-consuming anxiety, or a hormone imbalance. Often, a client's low libido is more likely to be a combination of all these factors than any given one. In other words, low libido is often a symptom of a larger issue, one that you have the power to address.

The BioEnergetic Model is tailored to exactly these types of situations; strengthening each BioEnergetic Element of your life will often address the issue of low libido at its root level, while also optimizing all those feel-good hormones that turn out to be oh-so-useful during sex. The result is an improvement in libido and sexual performance.

Of course, occasionally issues of sexual dysfunction may require a more specific, tailored approach, one that begins with testing to determine a personalized treatment plan. There are clinics across the country—including my own—which offer such an optimized approach.

For some people, there is still a bit of social embarrassment around seeking professional assistance for a low libido. So let me just say, there's a reason that sex goes in this category—Relationships—rather than simply in Exercise. Sex is often an important means of connection between partners; something that strengthens romantic relationships. Don't sell yourself short by ignoring your libido when you think about your overall health. Especially when the benefits of optimizing your libido can be so wonderful!

Oxytocin and Pets

Whether it's petting your own cat or dog, or a professionally trained therapy dog, this type of physical touch can increase oxytocin levels and decrease cortisol levels. Some people think of their furry friends as their "children," and so it makes sense that the oxytocin release is patterned on the mother-child relationship. Dog research, specifically with ancient Japanese breeds, but not wolves, demonstrated that elevated oxytocin secretion occurs in dogs, as well as their owners when they engage in a lot of eye contact.[182] Pre- and post-interaction oxytocin levels increased 130% in the dogs and 300% in their owners. Interspecies oxytocin release appears to be limited to dogs and humans and is likely related to canine domestication; similar outcomes have been reported in European dog breeds. (I know you were wondering about that.)

Building Your Community

To help explain why you need a community that helps you thrive, I'll use the gut microbiome as an analogy. The gut microbiome is the microbial community that lives synergistically within the gastrointestinal tract; it is comprised of what we think of as "good," or beneficial, bacteria and "bad," or pathogenic, bacteria. Microbiome researchers believe that having great diversity in the types of gut microorganisms is a good predictor of health, but at the same time, not all bad bacteria is bad. So, despite the presence

---

182   Miho Nagasawa et al., "Intranasal Oxytocin Treatment Increases Eye-Gaze Behavior toward the Owner in Ancient Japanese Dog Breeds," *Frontiers in Psychology* 8 (September 21, 2017): 1624.

of some bad bacteria, the good bacteria are quite capable of keeping the bad bacteria in check and preventing them from over-running the microbiome. The balance (homeostasis) created by and maintained by the good bacteria keeps us healthy. If a serious, life-threatening infection comes along for which an antibiotic is recommended, the bad bacteria strain can be successfully eradicated, and your body will overcome the trauma.

Similarly, we need to create and maintain healthy relationships within our social community. The goal is to have far more positive and nurturing relationships than negative ones. The beneficial relationships should fill the greatest volume in your community, and by including diverse relationships, you will thrive mentally and physically. At the same time, the risk of social isolation and all its health ramifications declines significantly.

So, if your crazy, antagonistic uncle is like the bad bacteria, you don't necessarily need to cut him out of your life entirely. Just minimize his influence by focusing on all the other positive influences in your life. Yet, if you are in an abusive relationship, it's like the life-threatening bacteria strain; in order to heal and move on, you need to take drastic action. If a toxic relationship is unsalvageable, first, acknowledge it is unfixable, and second, end it.

"May you reach that level within, where you no longer allow your past or people with toxic intentions to negatively affect or condition you."
—Lalah Delia

Good Communication Skills

Effective communication is critical to the success and survival of all relationships. The first step in being a good communicator is **active listening**. When you fully listen to another person, you are more likely to understand them, and from there, just about everything else is possible if you choose it to be. That sounds perfectly simple, but miscommunication and non-communication can be a great source of relationship strain and eventual failure.

"The most basic of all human needs is the need to understand and
be understood. The best way to understand people is to listen
to them."
—Ralph Nichols

Learning to communicate effectively is an ongoing process and a skill that can be difficult to master. But that being said, any relationship that's worth having is worthy of a sincere effort in advancing the relationship through effective communication. Here are five aspects to consider when interacting with another person face-to-face or on the phone (email and text are totally separate beasts):

1. *How did you say what you said?* – not just the actual words, but also your tone of voice (e.g., judgmental, unfeeling, mean or non-judgmental, empathetic).
2. *Why did you say what you said?* – your real intention (e.g., negative and to be hurtful or positive and to be helpful).
3. *What did you leave out?* – details that are left out may actually reveal more.
4. *When did you say it?* – saying things at an inopportune time (e.g., during an argument, as you walk out the door).
5. *What body language accompanied your words?* – your physical qualities that contradict or complement your words (e.g., facial expressions, posture, hand gestures).

"The most important thing in communication is hearing what
isn't said."
—Peter Drucker

The above quote by Peter Drucker reminds us that active listening and paying attention to non-verbal communication go hand-in-hand. While not every social engagement will attain this level of accomplishment, marital relationships and close friendships should aspire to it. Remember:

Communication is a two-way street, and relationships thrive when both parties are on board and communicate effectively. When you're developing your community, it's important to be yourself and to love yourself—others will follow.

Conclusion

Ultimately, improving the BioEnergetic Element of Relationships & Community requires something that most of my BioEnergetic Elements do not: courage. That's because community inevitably involves other people. You can change your nutrition, your exercise habits, your sleep patterns and even your meditation schedule without interacting with a single other human being. In fact, as COVID-19 quarantine experience has taught us, it can be surprisingly easy to go for weeks without any significant face-to-face interaction.

But relationships require interaction with others. And when other people get involved, things always get a little bit trickier: miscommunications arise, feelings get hurt, parents grow old, children grow up, friends move away or drift apart. Pain can result. It can be tough to be a social animal sometimes.

So, if you are by nature a bit shy or introverted, I want you to know that I get it. But ultimately, we are *social* animals. We were meant to live in groups. Our bodies were even designed that way—as our hormonal reaction to something as simple as a hug will demonstrate. When our relationships are strong our bodies respond on a biological level. And when our relationships are frayed, fractured, or deteriorated... our bodies still respond.

Once we understand this, we understand that our health is not a solo sport. There is only so much you can do by yourself to guarantee your own health. No amount of exercise will replace a broken or absent relationship. Instead, it is our strong connections to others that will help guarantee our health and longevity.

So, for your change-per-chapter, what is something you can implement tonight to better strengthen your relationships? It may be establishing a new greeting with a loved one, forgiving someone who hurt you, calling an old friend, resolving an argument, sending a gift, or responding to an email. Ultimately, any step that either builds positive relationships and social engagement or moves us away from social isolation or toxic relationships will be a good one.

5 to Thrive

1. There are numerous health benefits to being in a long-term, committed relationship, and these are increased when the relationship is a happy one.

2. Quality is more important than quantity when it comes to the mental health benefits of friendship.

3. Setting boundaries and putting distance between yourself and family members who encourage you to go into a Stress State is better than trying to force a family relationship that is unhealthy.

4. Loneliness is predictive of premature death and is particularly common in elderly people. This is a community concern and an area where you could do something positive for a community member.

5. Physical touch has a positive impact on the immune system and is now being used therapeutically in hospitals for a variety of purposes. For some of us, it can be uncomfortable or challenging to ask for affection and physical touch, but it does wonders for our physical and emotional wellbeing, so if you need one, ask for a hug!

For additional resources on elevating your relationships, visit thrivestate book.com/resources.

CHAPTER 10

REDISCOVERING YOUR SPIRIT AND PURPOSE

At one point or another in our lives, many of us question ourselves and our purposes. I'm not talking about the proverbial *mid-life crisis*, which is something completely different and has more to do with increasing age, perceived career or personal shortcomings, and inevitable mortality. I'm referring to a *crisis of undiscovered purpose*, which can happen to anyone regardless of age, yet similar to a mid-life crisis, it can produce feelings of anxiety, depression, and regret. Perhaps it's because we feel unfulfilled or unable to reach the untapped or underutilized talent deep within our being. Intuitively, we know it's there, but we just can't access what we can't put our finger on or define it in concrete, tangible terms. We ask, "Am I doing what I was meant to do?" or "Shouldn't I be doing something better for humanity?" or "Isn't there more to my life?"

PURPOSE is the seventh BioEnergetic Element, and it represents a nexus of the other six—sleep, nutrition, movement, stress/emotional mastery, mindset, and relationships—the spiritual element which elevates us to the ultimate Thrive State. We all belong to something bigger ("WE") than just our solitary selves ("ME").

"No man is an island entire of itself; every man is a piece of the continent, a part of the main; if a clod be washed away by the sea, Europe is the less, as well as if a promontory were, as well as any manner of thy friends or of thine own were; any man's death diminishes me, because I am involved in mankind. And therefore never send to know for whom the bell tolls; it tolls for thee."
—John Donne

It used to boggle me, and I would go into a state of analysis/paralysis wondering what my purpose was. But after deep research into epigenetics, understanding mind-body physiology, and learning from some spiritual teachers, the definition of purpose I've come up with is actually quite simple. Your purpose is YOU. Sharing YOU and your gifts with others is what you were made for. When you exit your mother's womb, you've made it; you've been chosen. We have been given talents, unique life experiences, and deep soul knowledge—and these are our gifts. Happiness and joy are our birthrights and encoded into our DNA. We see these traits in children all time. But sometimes we forget our joy and our gifts and are unable to express who we really are because we've picked up programs along the way—from our parents, culture, media, TV, and the environment (what Vishen Lakiani calls the culturescape)—which may steer us away from the life of joy, growth, and contribution we were meant to have. When we can remember who we authentically are and the things that spark joy and happiness in our lives, then share that with others, that's our purpose. Simple. But not always easy. My aim and sincere hope are for you to continue to take small, consistent action, just like you have in the previous chapters, to cultivate joy, love, and gratitude and give that gift of YOU to the world.

What Is Happiness?

Let's start with what happiness is and how we interpret it in our lives. When happiness is experienced in the here and now, it is a subjective human emotion within a current human experience. For example, you play competitive soccer, and your team wins its match; you (and your teammates) are happy in the current moment. You don't win every match, and when you lose, you feel something other than happiness. Overall, though, you feel happy because you have friends to play with (relationships and community), you are physically fit (movement), and you maintain balance in your life (stress and emotional control). Happiness in the broader sense of time becomes a subjective evaluation of life satisfaction or quality of life.

The keyword is *subjective*. Happiness depends on innumerable factors and is unique to each individual. What makes me happy may not make you happy, and vice versa. But how do you define happiness? The concepts of happiness and well-being have been debated since the days of ancient Greek philosophers who argued that the secret to a better and more harmonious life and thus, a better, more harmonious society, relied upon both virtuous character and eudaimonia. OK, so what the heck is *eudaimonia*, Dr. V?

Eudaimonia is a Greek word that commonly translates as "happiness" yet more likely approximates "human flourishing or prosperity" and "blessedness." Even from the ancient philosophical perspective, eudaimonia definitions differ. According to Aristotle, virtue and exercising virtue are central to eudaimonia, but also there is consideration given to external goods such as health, beauty, and wealth. Conversely (and for comparison), the Stoics did not believe external goods were necessary; for them, virtue was sufficient and necessary.

Aristotle believed that human beings gain eudaimonia when they develop their highest human functioning—rational thought and reason—and compliment these with rational actions. That's my super-condensed interpretation of Aristotle's meaning of eudaimonia. If you're interested in delving into the ancient origins of happiness and well-being, Aristotle's *Nicomachean Ethics* and the *Eudemian Ethics* are a good place to begin.

In my mind and for me personally, eudaimonia would be something like: I could have all the medical knowledge (reason), medical ability, and empathy for patients in the world, but if I don't put those qualities into action (work) by helping people, then I could not achieve true happiness. Put another way, when I fully participate in intellectually stimulating and fulfilling work for the benefit of others, then I have found my purpose, my happiness, and my success as a human being.

Eudaimonia, sometimes referred to as eudaimonic happiness, has a yin/yang counterpart, or an "evil twin" depending on how you look at it, called *hedonia* or hedonic happiness. Hedonia is the sense of happiness induced by momentary pleasure or satisfaction and immediate self-gratification. In my case, for example, hedonia could be the accolades of a colleague, a pay raise, or a new car (purchased because of the pay raise), all of which bring a sense of short-term happiness. No doubt that life brings a mix of hedonic and eudaimonic happiness, but what helps us achieve our purpose in life is the lasting happiness resulting from long-term goals and actions. Thus, the ideal human quest to achieve well-being is accomplished when we strive for meaning and a noble purpose and go beyond self-gratification.

Eudamonia in the 21st Century

Since the days of Aristotle, there has been a resurgence of interest in the concept of happiness, not by philosophers but by psychologists seeking to understand the effects on health. Most notably, Barbara L. Frederickson, a professor of psychology in the College of Arts and Sciences at the University of North Carolina at Chapel Hill, has put forth the ideas that (1) not all happiness is created equal; (2) that the human body recognizes this and responds differently; (3) eudaimonic happiness may provide health benefits at the cellular level; and (4) hedonic happiness may produce negative health effects at the cellular level. Wow, that's big! It means that two events seemingly equal in terms of eliciting a sense of happiness could, in fact, be experienced differently at the cellular level.

Epigenetic Influence

Dr. Frederickson's team collaborated with the team of Steven W. Cole, a professor of medicine, psychiatry, and behavioral sciences at the University of California at Los Angeles to examine how eudaimonic and hedonic well-being (happiness) influenced gene expression within human immune cells.[183] The premise was that when immune cells are under extended periods of stress or adversity, there is a shift in the normal gene expression; the fight-or-flight response activates something called the conserved transcriptional response to adversity (CTRA), which up-regulates pro-inflammatory genes and down-regulates genes involved in defending against viruses. Fifty-three genes were observed with respect to CTRA, including inflammation (19 genes), interferon response (31 genes), and antibody synthesis (3 genes). Although the participants as a whole reported feelings of well-being, those with high levels of hedonic well-being experienced a small increase in stress-related CTRA, and those with high levels of eudaimonic well-being experienced significant decreases in stress-related CTRA.

Dr. Fredrickson suggested that experiencing a greater amount of hedonic well-being is like consuming "empty calories." While simple pleasures may provide short-term gratification, they may cause long-term negative health effects. In other words, if you eat a whole pint of ice cream, you may feel good temporarily, but eating a pint every day will likely cause you to gain weight and could potentially lead to other poor health outcomes down the road. Dr. Cole states that eudaimonic well-being elicited a down-regulation of the pro-inflammatory genes' expression and an upregulation of the pro-immunity genes' expression. Put simply, having a strong sense of purpose will lower inflammation and increase immunity. As such, try to make eudaimonic happiness a priority in your life—your cells will reward you with good health, better performance, and greater healthspan. And with better health, performance, and healthspan, you'll have the power to continue sharing your talents and gifts with others who need them... and need you.

"At the cellular level, our bodies appear to respond better
to a different kind of well-being, one based on a sense of
connectedness and purpose."
—Barbara L. Fredrickson

---

183   Barbara L. Fredrickson et al., "A functional genomic perspective on human well-being," *Proceedings of the National Academy of Sciences of the United States of America* 110, no.33 (August 13, 2013): 13684-9.

Microbiome Influence

When the vast array of microorganisms inhabiting the gut microbiome are well cared for, physical and mental health flourish. The converse is also true. It is most certainly a mutualistic relationship; we take care of them, and they take care of us. Clinical research has demonstrated the connection between poor gut health and mental health challenges (e.g., anxiety, depression), but there's no strong evidence linking a healthy microbiome to eudaimonic well-being or happiness in general. In fact, research in this area is currently lacking, yet sure to be a focus in the future.[184] Due to the bidirectional connection between the gut and brain, I believe it is likely that a healthy and homeostatic gut microbiome could easily precipitate a sense of happiness. And because a sense of purpose lowers stress and inflammation as well as improves immunity, having purpose and eudaimonic happiness at least has an indirect role in promoting a healthy microbiome.

Telomere Influence

Chronic stress is a significant contributor to telomere shortening and degradation, and for many people, not experiencing eudaimonic well-being or finding their purpose in life can be quite stressful. When telomeres become too degraded, cells may die or become pro-inflammatory. Research comparing mothers caring for an autistic child (an extremely stressful job) with mothers caring for a non-autistic child found that the chronic stress elicited an elevated inflammatory response in peripheral blood mononuclear cells (PBMCs).[185] After fifteen months, the upregulation of pro-inflammatory genes was associated with shorter telomeres in PBMCs. This study and much of the current research is led by or influenced by Elizabeth H. Blackburn, PhD who co-discovered and won the 2009 Nobel Prize for

---

184   Gregor Reid, "Disentangling What We Know About Microbes and Mental Health," *Frontiers in Endocrinology* 10 (February 15, 2019): 81.

185   Jue Lin et al., "In vitro proinflammatory gene expression predicts in vivo telomere shortening: A preliminary study," *Psychoneuroendocrinology* 96 (October 2018): 179-187.

Physiology or Medicine with Carolyn W. Greider, PhD for telomerase, the enzyme which replenishes (lengthens) the telomere.

Dr. Blackburn co-authored *The Telomere Effect: A Revolutionary Approach to Living Younger, Healthier, Longer* with Elissa S. Epel, PhD in which they propose that we have the capability to improve our telomere health, thereby reducing the risk of some of the most common chronic diseases. Increasing resilience to stress via adequate sleep, good nutrition, regular exercise, meditation, social interaction, and long-term relationships—everything I've been talking about so far—is imperative to our telomeres and to reaching the Thrive State. And guess what else? Studies also show that those who have a greater sense of life purpose also have healthier telomeres. So, longer telomeres, improved cellular immunity, and decreased inflammation all happen from practicing eudaimonic happiness or having a sense of greater purpose. I don't know if you believe in higher power, but I sense our God, Source, or the Universe has created us in such a way to gift us with abundant health when we step into our power.

"Telomere science has grown into a clarion call.
It tells us that social stressors, especially as they affect children,
will result in exponentially higher costs down the line—
costs that are personal, physical, social, and economic.
You can respond to that call by, first, taking good care of yourself."
—Elizabeth H. Blackburn & Elissa S. Epel

Elements of Well-Being

Another well-known contemporary of Barbara Frederickson and Steven Cole is Carol D. Ryff, a professor of psychology at the University of Wisconsin at Madison, where she serves as director of the Institute on Aging. Dr. Ryff has identified six key elements of well-being, which are based on the principles of eudaimonia.[186] These include:

---

186   Carol D. Ryff , "Psychological well-being revisited: advances in the science and practice of eudaimonia," *Psychotherapy and Psychosomatics* 83, no.1 (2014): 10-28.

1. PURPOSE IN LIFE – having a sense of meaning and direction in one's life beyond life's small (hedonic) pleasures; purpose guides one's decisions and actions.

2. AUTONOMY – believing that one is living according to one's personal convictions and having the confidence to follow one's own path without worrying about what other people think.

3. PERSONAL GROWTH – exploring one's inner potential and making use of one's talents to pursue one's life purpose.

4. ENVIRONMENTAL MASTERY – learning to effectively navigate one's environment and manage life situations by utilizing one's internal resources (i.e., knowledge, skills) and external resources (i.e., tools, technology).

5. POSITIVE RELATIONSHIPS – having deep, meaningful connections with people who share similar life views.

6. SELF-ACCEPTANCE – having knowledge of one's personal limitations (and strengths) and being accepting of those weaknesses yet striving to improve oneself.

These six elements form the core of what it means to be human—to give meaning to our lives; to strive for something greater than ourselves; and to pursue the highest good within ourselves as Aristotle articulated more than two thousand years ago. Perhaps it is because we are living longer now than ever before in history and that our existence is more stable (for the most part), that understanding eudaimonic well-being has become more critical in advancing both mental and physical health and, ultimately, healthspan and human potential. As a physician, and one who believes that everyone is their best medicine, I advocate seeking eudaimonic well-being and happiness as a lifelong strategy to help patients overcome a wide array of health challenges related to chronic disease.

Rediscovering one's purpose in life is an integral part of well-being, and studies show that it's good for health. Here are a few research highlights from studies of aging American adults:

- Individuals with a high sense of purpose in life have a lower risk of cardiovascular events (e.g., heart attack, stroke) and of mortality due to any cause.[187]
- Adults over the age of 50 with a high sense of purpose in life maintain better physical function, such as walking speed and grip strength.[188]
- Individuals over the age of 50 with a high sense of purpose spend fewer nights in the hospital and are more likely to utilize preventive healthcare services (e.g., colonoscopy, mammogram, prostate exam).[189]
- There is sustained activation of the brain's reward circuitry in response to positive stimuli and lower cortisol secretion in adults with a high sense of purpose.[190]
- Alzheimer's patients with higher levels of purpose have more cognitive function while still alive than patients with lower levels of purpose despite similar brain pathology (i.e., amyloid plaque, tangles).[191]

Human Resilience

Have you ever known someone who seems to have encountered a lot of "bad luck" in life but always remained positive in the face of overwhelming adversity and managed to move forward? This person may struggle

---

187   Randy Cohen, Chirag Bavishi, and Alan Rozanski, "Purpose in Life and Its Relationship to All-Cause Mortality and Cardiovascular Events: A Meta-Analysis," *Psychosomatic Medicine* 78, no.2 (February – March 2016): 122-33.

188   Eric S. Kim et al., "Association Between Purpose in Life and Objective Measures of Physical Function in Older Adults," *JAMA Psychiatry* 74, no.10 (October 1, 2017): 1039-1045.

189   Eric S. Kim, Victor J. Strecher, and Carol D. Ryff, "Purpose in life and use of preventive health care services," *Proceedings of the National Academy of Sciences of the United States of America* 111, no.46 (November 18, 2014): 16331-6.

190   Carol D. Ryff et al., "Purposeful Engagement, Healthy Aging, and the Brain," *Current Behavioral Neuroscience Reports* 3, no.4 (December 2016): 318–327.

191   Patricia A. Boyle et al., "Effect of Purpose in Life on the Relation Between Alzheimer Disease Pathologic Changes on Cognitive Function in Advanced Age," *Archives of General Psychiatry* 69, no.5 (May 2012): 499-505.

in life, but no one would ever know it unless they knew that person's life circumstances. This may well be due to possessing a strong sense of one's purpose in life. A current hypothesis is that purpose promotes resilience (homeostasis) by regulating the potentially negative emotional response elicited by stressful or unpleasant events. In other words, an individual with a higher level of purpose would reframe a negative event into a positive event (a challenge, opportunity), and thus, not subject his/her cells to the ill effects of increased cortisol and other stress-related hormones. Having purpose involves looking at the world with a wide-angle lens to get a more encompassing view of everything around us, rather than a narrowly focused, or even obstructed, view.

In Chapter 8: Mindset Is Everything, you learned how our consciousness, our new choices, and repeated intentional actions have the power to shift and change our disempowering subconscious beliefs and old neuronal wiring through neuroplasticity. It is through neuroplasticity—our ability to form new neural connections—that human resilience can be trained, in that very space that Victor Frankl describes: "where we have the power to choose our response."

> "Our greatest glory is not in never falling,
> but in rising every time we fall."
> —Confucius

Don't Worry, Be Happy.

OK, OK. Go ahead and start singing the tune. It'll put a smile on your face— even if you're having a lousy day. Grammy Award winner Bobby McFerrin, Jr. was on to something with his 1988 hit song and the countless smiles it created. Eudaimonic happiness and well-being are essential to one's inner spirit—your inner being, soul, or whatever term you use to describe that within you which gives you emotional and intellectual energy. Consider these "virtues" as instruments to compliment your inner spirit as you journey towards your purpose:

- Know thyself (the "real" you).
- Trust your body, your instincts, and your inner desires.
- Release your authentic self.
- Live fully engaged with the world around you.
- Learn to forgive.
- Practice gratitude.

Now do me a favor. Take out a piece of paper and answer the following five questions with as many items you can think of. Take as much time as you need to completely and honestly address each question; you can set it aside for an hour, or a day, and come back to it with a fresh perspective after you've had some time to let your thoughts percolate. When you're satisfied with your list, move on to the action plan.

THE HAPPINESS LIST
1. *What makes you happy?*
2. *Who are the people that bring the most happiness and joy to your life right now?*
3. *What activities spark joy in your life right now?*
4. *Is there something you used to do in the past that made you happy that you no longer do?*
5. *Is there someone or something keeping you from being truly happy?*

THE HAPPINESS ACTION PLAN
1. *Based on your answers on the happiness list, what change(s) do you need to make in order to be happier? As always, start with the easiest change to implement.*
2. *Make a commitment to yourself to increase the happiness in your life.*
**OPTIONAL: Set a timeline to implement the changes you indicated in #1.

The Power of Being Thankful

Gratitude (noun): the quality of being thankful; a strong feeling of appreciation towards someone who has demonstrated kindness towards you. Gratitude also means being appreciative and satisfied with what you presently have, not what you lack (or what you think you lack). When people are grateful, they acknowledge the goodness in their lives and in doing so are able to connect to something bigger than themselves and find purpose.

In the same way that forgiveness benefits the giver and receiver, so does gratitude, and both these experiences find their origins and focus in religion, philosophy, and more recently, psychology. Having a sense of gratitude can promote short-term happiness (an in-the-moment experience) or long-term happiness (life satisfaction). Conversely, resentment is associated with life dissatisfaction. Studies examining the effects of gratitude meditation on mental well-being found greater neural connectivity in the emotion-regulating areas of the brain as well as lower heart rates.[192] Because stress, anger, and resentment are common components of daily life, researchers believe that if individuals utilize daily gratitude meditation, they will be better equipped to manage stress, control negative emotions, and enhance self-motivation, thereby improving life satisfaction and sense of happiness.

Additional health benefits of expressing gratitude include:

- Expressing gratitude (i.e., consciously focusing on one's blessings) promotes a positive mindset and reduces perceived stress levels.[193]
- Individuals who are grateful are more empathetic and generous and are less aggressive; this is especially true in people who express gratitude towards a parent. Cultivating a sense of gratitude promotes mental

---

192 Sunghyon Kyeong et al., "Effects of gratitude meditation on neural network functional connectivity and brain-heart coupling," *Scientific Reports* 7, no.11 (July 2017): 5058.

193 Robert A. Emmons and Michael E. McCullough, "Counting blessings versus burdens: an experimental investigation of gratitude and subjective well-being in daily life," *Journal of Personality and Social Psychology* 84, no.2 (February 2003): 377-89.

well-being, improves interpersonal relationships, and benefits society through the reduction of aggression.[194]

- Older adults who engage in simple gratitude exercises daily experience less loneliness and, in turn, improved health.[195]
- High school students engaging in weekly gratitude writing exercises improve their healthy eating behaviors.[196]

A 2016 study also evaluated the role of optimism in patients with acute coronary syndrome (ACS).[197] ACS (heart attack and/or unstable angina) is a significant cause of hospital admissions and frequently leads to rehospitalization or death within the following year. Patients were evaluated on post-ACS physical activity levels, inflammatory biomarkers, and rehospitalization. Optimism was associated with greater physical activity levels and fewer hospital readmissions in the subsequent six months.

Gratitude is experienced in the present moment by focusing on past and current events (e.g., "I am grateful to be alive." or "I am grateful for my family."), whereas optimism is experienced by focusing on future expectations (e.g., "My future health will be better." or "I will exercise more in the future to prevent another ACS."). Even though optimism may be more action-based than gratitude, both are important for well-being. Perhaps, the lesson is that when you practice gratitude, you will be more optimistic about your future health, which will lead to positive health behaviors like good nutrition, exercise, sleep, stress management, positive mindset, nurturing relationships, and purpose.

---

194   C. Nathan DeWall et al., "A Grateful Heart is a Nonviolent Heart: Cross-Sectional, Experience Sampling, Longitudinal, and Experimental Evidence," *Social Psychological and Personality Science* 3 (2012): 232–240.

195   Monica Y. Bartlett and Sarah N. Arpin, "Gratitude and Loneliness: Enhancing Health and Well-Being in Older Adults," *Research on Aging* 41, no.8 (September 2019): 772-793.

196   Megan M. Fritz et al., "Gratitude facilitates healthy eating behavior in adolescents and young adults," *Journal of Experimental Social Psychology* 81 (2019): 4-14.

197   Jeff C. Huffman, "The Effects of Optimism and Gratitude on Physical Activity, Biomarkers, and Readmissions Following an Acute Coronary Syndrome: The Gratitude Research in Acute Coronary Events (GRACE) Study," *Circulation: Cardiovascular Quality and Outcomes* 9, no.1 (January 2016): 55-63.

Be Grateful... Every Day

Sure, that sounds simple enough, but for a great many people, being grateful requires practice. Building gratitude is just like building muscle. You've got to set your mind to it and work at it. Even on the days when you wake up feeling as if you have little or nothing to be grateful for, dig a little deeper, and I'm sure you will find something or someone for which you can express gratitude. And just like muscles, it's *use it or lose* it for gratitude, too.

> **Dr. V's PURPOSE Rx:**
> Apply the same commitment to practicing gratitude every day as you do to daily exercise.

Cultivating Gratitude

- Write down whatever or whomever makes you feel grateful (gratitude journaling).
- Write thank-you notes.
- Tell someone you are grateful for them or thank them for their kindness.
- Provide a random act of kindness to a stranger.
- Focus your meditation or prayer on whatever or whomever you are grateful for.
- Freely share your gift with your community.

> *"The best way to find yourself is to lose yourself*
> *in service to others."*
> —Mahatma Gandhi

Service to Others

Earlier in this book, I talked about how every cell in our body must work as part of a larger collective. This is the core principle of purpose—contributing our gifts to the larger collective (I'll say more about this in Chapters 11 and 12). A cell that decides to live only for itself is a cancerous cell, replicating and growing without any heed for the consequences. Well, we, too, are part of a collective, a community. We are cells within the colossal body of our collective humanity. Are we doing our part to keep this body alive? Or are we living only for ourselves?

We each have a role to play, but this role is aligned not with our bank account or our job title; it is based on our passion and purpose. Finding our spirit, our joy, and our gifts and sharing them with others through service completes us and helps the entire community thrive alongside us. This is why we were chosen to be blessed with this life. When the selfish "ME" transforms into the selfless "WE," then we are truly fulfilling our role on this Earth.

For me, this drive to transform "ME" into "WE" inspired me to found the Live Again Project in late 2016. The Live Again Project was a sponsored nonprofit that helped connect and transform the world through the stories of terminal cancer patients, just like Ishmael. With the Live Again Project, these patients—or their loved ones—shared their hope and dreams, their reflections, and their life lessons. In a lot of ways, the Live Again Project was an extension of my experience with Ishmael: a terminal cancer patient had changed my life with only a few words, after all. *What other lives can be changed through the power of such a story?* I wondered.

But beyond that, in my interventional radiology work I had seen how completely people's priorities can shift upon receiving a cancer diagnosis. I had noticed that those who fixated on the injustice of their diagnosis—and fairly so, of course—remained in a bitter state during the course of their treatment, often unable to let go of their anger and resentment at the misfortune that had befallen them. Other patients were able to make a conceptual shift, to instead focus on the question of what they were going to do with their remaining time. And, in my personal perception, it was the latter group of patients who responded better overall to their treatments.

I believe that this type of reflection, this type of questioning—*What do I want with my remaining time on this Earth? What are my goals now that mortality is staring me in the face? How do I want to show up?* —is intimately connected to the stories we tell ourselves and others about our identity and about our stories. Storytelling doesn't cure cancer, but I do believe that storytelling helps.

It has been my hope that, with the Live Again Project, we can inspire others to tell their—and their loved ones'—stories, to share their emotions and their reflections in a safe and supportive community, and to build a space for conversation and healing. With Live Again, we are telling people that cancer does not get to tell their story; they do. Finally, by sharing the stories of these patients, we share their impact and carry on their legacy in two very important ways: (1) First, they inspire others with their courage and character. They show us the best of humanity in an unthinkable situation, and so challenge the rest of us to become better humans in whatever our situation may be. (2) Second, we identify the charities and projects they love and find ways to support those causes, financially or otherwise, so that even if cancer wins the battle, it never wins the war.

There are other ways that I have endeavored, personally, to be of service to others—beyond my direct work with patients, that is. I speak and write about the great work being done in various health fields—as you well know since you're reading my book! I consider myself a bit of a health evangelist, sharing the news about medical advances that may hold the key to increasing human healthspan and making our lives better—genomics, molecular imaging, novel oncologic therapies, health empowerment, alternative therapies, biohacking, the epigenetics of purpose, community, laughter, forgiveness, and gratitude. And while I still practice medicine, I've added elements to my practice to focus on empowering patients and people to become their own best medicine, even if they're not "sick" by the traditional definition.

I believe all of us are capable of turning ME into WE. We are all here for a purpose, and now more than ever, the world needs us to become the heroes within. I'm on a mission to create a world free of disease and to empower you not only to discover not only your healing powers but also to *re*-discover your own

> Dr. V's PURPOSE Rx: Keep an inventory of the things, people, and activities you do that spark joy in your life. Then share that joy with others.

joyful and authentic self. My desire is for you to live a long and happy life and perform at your very best and to show you that the world can fully appreciate your gifts. Your purpose is YOU. Rediscover what brings you joy and happiness, your gift, and give it away to others. I invite you to be a part of our growing movement of health and fun seekers determined to live, laugh, and love more courageously. Join me in this journey to health, and let's create a better world together.

5 to Thrive

1. Your purpose is YOU. Sharing YOU and your gifts (talents, joy, life experiences) with others is what you were made for.

2. Eudaimonia is happiness which encompasses a sense of purpose in one's life. This type of happiness has been shown to have benefits at the cellular level, including decreased inflammation, improved cellular immunity, and better telomere health.

3. Gratitude leads to greater overall happiness, but it takes practice. Try journaling or writing thank-you cards as a tangible expression of gratitude.

4. Rediscovering your purpose is more a process of active remembering, rather than of active looking or seeking. Remembering that we have been chosen, and that we are enough. Remembering that joy and happiness is our birthright. Remembering that life is a gift and that we've been given gifts to share.

5. Be You. Do You. Share You. #YOUIT #YouAreYourBestMedicine

CHAPTER 11

THE THRIVE STATE ADVANTAGE: GOING FROM ME TO WE

During the COVID pandemic, I had the opportunity to give keynotes and workshops to executives from businesses, including Whole Foods, Bank of America, Walgreens, CVS Pharmacy, Morgan Stanley, and Varsity Healthcare Partners, as well as non-profits such as GoodDays.org and the Live Again Project. As I became more involved with these organizations, I was able to see parallels between the health and functioning of the human body and the health and functioning of organizations.

The human body and organizations are both ecosystems—interconnected systems that share common traits: independence, interdependence, and state dependence. That is to say, every constituent within the ecosystem plays their own independent role in the system; that role is necessary for the survival of the ecosystem; and the state of the ecosystem affects everything in it. Take for example the ecosystem of an aquarium, pond, or lake. The aquatic plants in that ecosystem provide the oxygen for all the fish, and the herbivorous fish nibble on the plants. The fish release carbon dioxide which then combines with the sun's rays for photosynthesis within plants' chloroplasts. If all components are available, the ecosystem is balanced and in a great state. But, if for some reason the state of the ecosystem is disturbed—the temperature drops precipitously, or there's no sunlight around, or a toxic chemical is dumped into the water—then every living species in that ecosystem suffers. (I'm simplifying things here, of course—ecosystems, like human bodies, are incredibly complex.)

Or think about another (very simplified) ecosystem: a national economy. In an economy, employers pay workers wages for their labor. Those workers use their wages to purchase goods and services from companies. Those companies use that income to pay their own workers, so they, too, can buy goods and services from other companies. Companies and workers both pay taxes to the government, which provides services such as public safety, roads and bridges, allowing workers and goods to move around and interact safely. Companies, too, buy and make goods and services for each other, generating even more economic activity. All of this activity is considered healthy. So long as all the components are healthy and both supply and demand are balanced, things run smoothly. But if something changes—for example, some companies are mismanaged and go out of business, costing workers their jobs, or some workers go on strike and decide not to work anymore—then the entire economy can suffer. And similarly, the state of the economy affects everything in it - think of interest rates, various markets, etc.—during the state of bull or bear markets.

The Human Body as an Ecosystem

Because of interdependence, every cell in the body must do its job well (independence) for the benefit of the entire system. Take, for example, what would happen if a lung cell was 5% less efficient in extracting oxygen from the inhaled air. All of sudden, the rest of the body's cells would receive less of this vital nutrient. In turn, this would make every cell and every organ less optimal. As a consequence, there would be more toxins and metabolic waste in the body due to suboptimal liver and kidney cells; poorer circulation due compromised heart cells; and, of course, this would make the original lung cell perform even more poorly than its original state of non-peak performance.

You can see what happens with an interconnected and interdependent ecosystem; when one cell is not pulling its weight, the entire ecosystem suffers. An optimized ecosystem is one in which every single member reaches and performs at their highest potential. As a reminder, the Thrive State is the state of optimal health, longevity, and peak performance. Through our conscious choices, we create epigenetic messages to our DNA giving them signals to either Thrive or Survive. In the Thrive State, every individual cell is performing at their best while serving the entire system (i.e., cells live in service to the whole). Conversely, in the Stress State, cells are merely surviving, which leads to suboptimal performance, chronic system failure, and eventually chronic disease. Cells that are not at their best cannot serve the entire system (i.e., cells live in service to themselves). A well-known example of when a cell—and other cells along with it—goes rogue is cancer.

The Organization as an Ecosystem

Organizations work much the same way. Human beings in organizations are like cells in the human body. Instead of forming organs, human beings gather together in teams and departments, which are interdependent and have symbiotic and synergistic relationships amongst themselves. This allows the entire organization to thrive. For example, the research and development department creates an excellent product or service, which relies on the marketing department to advertise and distribute, the sales team to sell, and customer service department to keep customers happy. Then there's the operations department that makes sure workflows are optimized; financial department to make sure there's always a cash flow; and an information system department to facilitate communication. And last, but not least, an executive team that oversees everything. If any one of these departments functions poorly, the entire organization will be affected. If even one person in a department is functioning less than optimally, that is going to compromise the optimal effectiveness of that department.

You can see why I started to draw Thrive State parallels between human beings and organizations, can't you?

ECOSYSTEM OF THE BODY

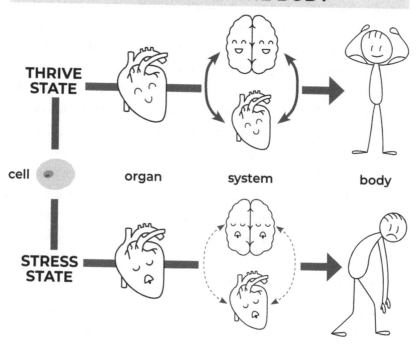

ECOSYSTEM OF THE ORGANIZATION

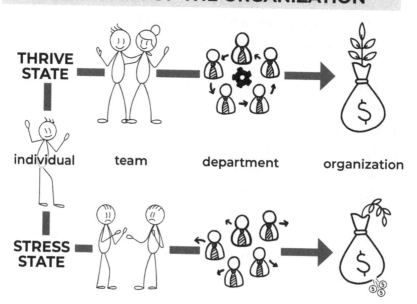

Pressure - the Growth Opportunity of an Ecosystem

Every so often, some force—pressure—challenges the fabric of human ecosystems—our bodies, our teams, and our organizations.

On January 20, 2020, a cruise ship named the Diamond Princess departed Yokohama, Japan. Five days later, an 80-year-old man requiring medical attention disembarked. His cough and fever turned out to be COVID pneumonia. The entire cruise ship was quarantined for 27 days. This isolated outbreak aboard the Diamond Princess represents a social experiment we can't do realistically or ethically: put hundreds of people together in close quarters, expose them to a novel and contagious virus, and wait to see what happens. Ultimately, one in five people aboard became infected, and 2% of those infected died. Unknown to this day are the even larger numbers of people who survived but continue to experience debilitating symptoms.

People worldwide experienced the pressure of the subsequent pandemic not only personally, but also on their organizations and businesses. Many experienced and are continuing to experience tumultuous drops in the physical and mental health, morale, and productivity of their workforce. In late 2022, Gallup announced that at least 50% of workers are either "quietly quitting" or not engaged with their organizations. Across the spectrum, businesses are struggling to hire and keep good people.

These findings bring up some important questions.

1. Why do some people suffer from severe and even fatal forms of an infectious illness, yet others experience only mild symptoms or none at all?
2. Similarly, why do some organizations have employees that routinely quit on them, while others are a magnet for attracting and keeping the best people?
3. How are some people and organizations able to access optimal health, longevity, and peak performance no matter how challenging the situation?
4. How do people and organizations have the physical, mental, emotional, and spiritual fortitude to remain resilient in the face of change?

5. Is there one quality that allows for people and organizations to thrive under pressure and change, while others barely survive?

I can answer the last question first. After directly working with and learning from the highest performing and longest living humans and organizations, I see the one common trait that separates these individuals and organizations that thrive versus others that are merely surviving: Optimized Human Potential.

If you recall, our human bodies encompass all the genes and gifts inherited from the many generations of natural selection preceding us. The Thrive State, almost by definition, is the state of being that activates our human potential. Remember, our biological machinery is equipped with an immune system that protects us from the tiniest of pathogens. We have been gifted with the mental acuity and innovation to put a man on the moon and create a supercomputer that can fit in our pocket; the emotional intelligence to create great works of music and art; and a physical body capable of scaling the world's tallest mountains and surfing the largest waves.

The COVID pandemic has shown people that mere survival is not enough. There's been a paradigm shift in people's values. People now expect more out of themselves and the people they work with. And instead of being susceptible to the next lurking stress or disaster, they want to be empowered by the knowledge, the tools, and the organizations that will help them thrive.

> "The healthier an organization is, the more of its intelligence
> it is able to tap into and use. Most organizations exploit
> only a fraction of the knowledge, experience, and intellectual
> capital that is available to them. But the healthy ones
> tap into almost all of it."
> —Patrick Lencioni

Patrick Lencioni is one of the founders of The Table Group and is the pioneer of the organizational health movement. As he describes, "An organization has integrity—is healthy—when it is whole, consistent, and complete, that is, when its management, operations, strategy, and culture fit together and make sense." With a similar definition, the McKinsey Global Institute states organizational health is the "ability to align around and achieve strategic goals." Prior to the COVID-19 pandemic, these were common definitions of organizational health.

The gift of the pandemic allowed for a renewed focus and attention on the physical, mental, emotional, social, and spiritual aspects of health and human potential. In 2020, McKinsey published "Prioritizing health: A prescription for prosperity" which offers an excellent rationale for organizations and businesses to adopt BioEnergetic enhancement strategies in the workplace: "Improving health has the potential to be a societal and economic game changer. After all, few investments deliver against so many of today's social needs, substantially improving well-being and reducing inequity, while also delivering an impressive shot in the arm to the global economy—and all with a high return on investment."

Long past are the days of conventional occupational health and safety. Although on-the-job health and safety are important, the "unhealth" of workers and companies is increasingly influenced by lack of sleep, increased sedentariness, and mental health stressors. Research from the McKinsey Global Institute also shows that "70% of actions to improve health happen before a sick patient seeks care. Half of that comes from living in healthier environments, societies, and workplaces that encourage healthy behaviors and mindsets. Long-term prevention and health promotion cannot simply be left to health care providers or health care systems. It is quite literally everybody's business. And just plain good business at that."[198]

---

198 Jaana Remes and Shubham Singhal, "Good health is good business. Here's why," *Fortune* (July 9, 2020).

REAL LIFE EXAMPLES OF THRIVING WORKPLACES

- Middlesbrough Environment City (MEC), a small British charity organization, implemented a health and well-being program which included aspects to address the BioEnergetic Elements of nutrition, movement, and stress. Team-building activities improved relationships among employees and improved morale. Employees' overall health improved, and the organization benefited with a decrease in the annual sick-day rate—from 4.25 days to 2.4 days.[199]

- Digital Outlook Communications, a London-based digital marketing and creative agency, employed several BioEnergetic initiatives—supported by senior management—to successfully address its "long hours culture." In a two-year period, absenteeism improved 95%, from 4 days per employee to 0.22 days. Staff turnover decreased from 34% to 9%, and the company reaped the cost-saving benefits from recruitment and training expenses.[200]

- Several of BMW's production plants retrofitted their production lines to be more ergonomic, thereby reducing physical stress for older workers. A strength and stretching exercise program was also introduced. In the first year of implementation, BMW achieved a 7% improvement in productivity, and the productivity of older workers equaled that of younger workers. Absenteeism fell from 7% to 2% in just one year.[201]

---

199 "Case study: Middlesbrough Environment City - healthy eating and exercise 2013," Department for Work & Pensions, www.gov.uk/government/case-studies/middlesbrough-environment-city-healthy-eating-and-exercise.

200 "Business in the Community. Healthy People = Healthy Profits," London: 2009.

201 Christopher Loch et al., "The Globe: How BMW is Defusing the Demographic Time Bomb," *Harvard Business Review* (March 2010).

It is the collective optimized human potential that allows organizations to be more productive, collaborative, innovative, and resilient. When these organizations cultivate this potential in each member and show that everyone is valued, they are in turn, able to attract, engage, and keep the best people.

The energetic state of an organization and its effect on organizational performance is not a novel concept. In 2011, Heike Bruch and Bernd Vogel published *Fully Charged: How Great Leaders Boost Their Organization's Energy and Ignite High Performance*. They suggest organizational leadership has a significant role to play in facilitating (or diminishing) their company's collective energetic state.[202] The task of energetic state management of the people within organizations should be tailored to the specific needs of the department, team, or group; if it's possible, addressing the energetic state of the individual yields additional benefit.

Bruch and Vogel describe four different energetic states that could potentially exist within an organization. They are noteworthy because they characterize most organizations to some degree, predict an organization's productivity and growth metrics, and can lead to conflicts of varying intensity and duration which may impact the organization's effectiveness.

Productive Energy	Comfortable Energy
• Channeled emotions & effort towards common goals • Collective enthusiasm & focus	• High satisfaction & feeling of ease with the status quo • Potential for complacency
Resigned Inertia	**Corrosive Energy**
• Mental withdrawal or indifference towards company's goals • Low energy & decreased ability for change, innovation, and performance	• High levels of anger & distrust • Potential for internal conflicts • May result in damage to strategy or projects

202   Heike Bruch and Bernd Vogel, *Fully Charged: How Great Leaders Boost Their Organization's Energy and Ignite High Performance* (Massachusetts: Harvard Business School Publishing, 2011).

Although Bruch and Vogel didn't consider the physical, mental, emotional, social, and spiritual components of these energetic states, I know YOU, the reader of Thrive State, can see how these bioenergetic elements influence the energetic state of ecosystems.

To review this chapter thus far, a team, organization, or business is an ecosystem just like the human body. These ecosystems share three common traits: independence, interdependence, and state dependence. The Thrive State is the energetic state of optimized human potential which activates the biology of optimal health, longevity, and peak performance in the human body, and extends these benefits into organizations which lead to improved productivity, performance, and prosperity.

If you belong to larger ecosystem such as a family, team, or organization, you may want to consider the following questions:

1. How does your organization support the needs of the bioenergetic elements for each of their constituents—sleep, nutrition, movement, emotional, mental, social, and spiritual?

2. Are optimal health, longevity, and peak performance core values for your organization?

3. Across the Thrive and Survive state spectrum, what is the current state of your organization? What is the current state of your organization's health, productivity, morale, teamwork, innovation, and impact in the local communities and the larger world?

4. If nothing was done to change the current state of your organization, what would it be missing out on? What possibilities would be lost due to underperforming potential?

5. What new reality is possible with your organization when it has an optimized workforce, teams, and teamwork?

Cultivating the Thrive State in Teams, Communities, and Organizations

I often get asked how one can start implementing the Thrive State into their organization. The good news is, you don't need to have anything else other than the principles in this book to begin. And as a reminder, it starts with choice. Your conscious choices that lead to actions and habits will create the state in your body and your immediate surroundings. It's great if you're the CEO and would like create a new culture or initiative within your company, but ANYONE, any one—no matter what gender, job title, sex, race, or status—can positively affect the state of a group, an organization, an environment, and even the planet simply by changing the state within themselves first. Gandhi did say, "Be the change you want to see in the world."

When we elevate our state, we not only change the message we give to our cells, but others feel it as well. Most species on this planet, especially humans, have evolved with the biological machinery to thrive in community. Our genetic code—telomeres, CTRA, epigenetic clocks—informs us that community and purpose activate the biology of human potential. We are equipped to be able to communicate through language, yes, but we also are wirelessly interconnected to communicate. One such biological system is mirror neurons.

Mirror neurons were first discovered in the early 1990s, when a team of Italian researchers found individual neurons in the brains of macaque monkeys that fired both when the monkeys grabbed an object and also when the monkeys watched another primate grab the same object. Essentially, mirror neurons respond to actions that we observe in others. In addition to imitation and learning, they are responsible for a myriad of other sophisticated human behavior and thought processes. Mirror neurons respond both when perceiving an action and while executing an action. They provide a direct internal experience of another person's actions or emotions and may be the neurological basis of empathy. Our bodies also have other detection systems to feel someone else's scowl or smile; be transported through different emotional states through sounds or music; and likely also have receptors that detect small subtle shifts in energy beyond our five conscious known senses. Have you ever walked into a space and without seeing or hearing anything, feel the mood or energy it exudes? Some people call this intuition.

The process of transforming my own Stress State into the Thrive State involved truly accepting and loving every part of me, including every single cell that does its part to give me this amazing life. This is true for thriving organizations as well. It is because of these interconnected systems that make change—good or bad—spread through ecosystems and organizations so quickly. One could easily spread fear across an ecosystem or business as quickly as someone can spread good. Just like the choice of creating the Thrive State in your body begins with your decision and commitment, the Thrive State in organizations is achieved when one or a few leaders commit to act, to live, and to be the example of what they want to see in their organizations. YES, I will talk about love in the organizational setting. Do you love every single member or your organization? Can you see the best in everyone even when they don't yet see it within themselves? Does your workforce feel like your organization has their best interest at heart and is looking out for them and their families?

One such example of how one person's state can transform a community and business is my late dear brother and mentor, Eric "The Trainer" Fleishman, who built a fitness and media empire. You may remember him from the Movement Chapter. He unexpectedly passed on Thanksgiving Day in 2022.

Eric treated every person he encountered exactly the same, whether they were an A-list celebrity or on the waitlist for government assistance. Eric wouldn't let two people enter a room without highlighting the brightness and talents of each of them as they met for the first time. He saw the best in people and made sure everyone saw themselves as the beautiful human beings they are. He was such a generous and giving person, with an uplifting and service-first mentality. Yes, the Thrive State started with Eric, but his energy transformed it into a culture, a way of being and treating others, that radiated to every employee, every client, and every initiative he took on, whether it be a charity event, TV or movie project, or eight- and nine-figure business deals. Because of this Thrive State culture, Eric was always a magnet for clients, employees, endorsements, and new business. It is also because of this culture that his clients and employees have remained loyal and engaged, no matter the season.

When the pandemic forced gym shutdowns in California, Eric didn't stress about lost revenue, instead he went back to his modus operandi of *Who Can I Help?* So, he created a free online workout show called Eric the Trainer (ETT) Live where he would lead people through an entertaining workout and would frequently invite celebrity guests on to interview—it was like Bootcamp meets the Tonight Show. He made it completely free, without thought of a business plan or revenue streams. He just chose to serve people the best way he knew how—blending fitness with entertainment. After the pandemic, ETT Live turned into a lucrative online fitness platform which attracted users and sponsors from all over the world.

When Eric's passing was announced to the public a few days later, there was an outpouring of love and messages from all around the world—from the celebrities he trained, to heads of fitness companies, executives from Mr. Olympia and Mr. America pageants, and everyday people who had a chance to meet him at an event or on the street. Tens of thousands of messages, all with a similar theme: "Most positive guy I met." "Helped me in my darkest moments." "Believed in me and my dreams before I did." "His vibrant energy and generosity are contagious." "He helped me connect with the strongest parts of myself." I hope these comments give you a sense of who this person was. It reminds me of Maya Angelou's famous quote: "People will forget what you said, people will forget what you did, but people will never forget how you made them feel." He was the true embodiment of Thrive State.

Eric's company optimized components of a Thriving Ecosystem: Independence, Interdependence, and State Dependence. Independence: Every individual was treated with love, respect, and encouraged and nurtured to become the best version of themselves. Interdependence: Everyone sought to become a better version of themselves so they could serve their gifts to others. State Dependence: By living, breathing, and optimizing the bioenergetic elements—by being the Thrive State—everyone in the ecosystem had the aptitude to perform at their best and be resilient against outside pressure. By living Thrive State principles, every member of the ETT Enterprise transformed the pressure of the pandemic into growth— not only physically, mentally, emotionally, socially, and spiritually, but also financially and at an enterprise level as well.

The Thrive State Advantage

People ask me what type of results organizations can expect from being in the Thrive State—from optimizing the physical, mental, emotional, social, and spiritual energetics of the ecosystem. Let's just isolate one component for now—Emotional. Have you heard about the Happiness Advantage?

Former Harvard researcher and current positive psychology corporate trainer Shawn Anchor introduces the concept of happiness and its effect on organizations. He challenges the popular—yet completely inaccurate— notions regarding the "formula for success" that we've been following since childhood. First school, and later the workplaces, teach us that *if I work harder, I will be more successful. If I'm more successful, then I'll be happier.* In this model, the goalposts for happiness are continually moving, and the brain simply doesn't work that way. Instead, Shawn promotes raising the positivity level in the present, which the brain experiences as a Happiness Advantage. This leads to increases in creativity, intelligence, energy levels, and improvements in measurable business outcomes. According to Shawn, "The greatest competitive advantage in the modern economy is a positive and engaged brain." Of course, happy employees will also benefit; they're less stressed, less prone to burnout, and better at keeping their jobs (i.e., job security).

The Happiness Advantage for Businesses:[203]

- 31% higher productivity
- 37% higher sales
- 19% higher accuracy
- 50% greater revenues
- Up to 10x more employee engagement

These are the results of just improving one of the 7 bioenergetic elements. Imagine the results if the other six bioenergetic elements were also optimized.

Thrive State Activates More Flow

Some of the bioenergetic elements are actually flow triggers, so therefore being in the Thrive State leads to more episodes of flow. "Flow" is defined as an optimal state of consciousness which allows us to feel our best and perform our best. It's akin to the concept of "being in the zone." Originally, flow was associated with peak performance in athletes, but today, flow has become a sought-after state by entrepreneurs and professionals of every stripe. Steven Kotler, Executive Director of Flow Research Collective, offers a compelling argument as to why we can and should strive to be in a state of flow. Foremost, Kotler believes that every individual has a "built-in" state of flow that is a by-product of human evolution and when accessed, it amplifies performance. Being in a state of flow also increases creativity, which is integral to problem solving and talent expression (i.e., art, music, dance, writing, technology, etc.).

When employees achieve a Flow State, they're able to unlock their peak mental performance which in turn, increases the organization's bottom line. Organizational benefits include retaining top talent, improving productivity,

---

203   "Happiness Fuels Success," The Happiness Advantage | Orange Frog Workshop™, www .orangefrogenterprise.com/training2022.

and increasing innovation and impact. Individual benefits include better mental health, less burnout, and increased life satisfaction. In fact, people with the most flow have the most life satisfaction, and this ultimately leads to happiness—a great reason to focus on optimizing your flow state. When labor becomes passion, individuals and organizations reap the benefits.

Exponential Results when Employees are in Flow:[204]

- Top executives who are in flow are 5x (500%) more productive than those who are out of flow.
- Employees who spend 2 workdays in flow are 10x (1000%) more productive than the competition who spend 5 workdays in non-flow.
- Flow amplifies creativity by 4-7x (400-700%) versus those who are out of flow.

If being in the Flow State is ideal, how exactly do you get there? Kotler and others in the field of peak performance have suggested that there are individual and group triggers which encourage the brain to release certain neurochemicals that prime your body or your organization for flow. Group flow triggers, which are important in an organization or business setting include: shared goals; close listening; complete concentration; equal participation; open communication; blending egos; a sense of control; familiarity; shared risk; moving forward ("yes, and..."). I would add to this by saying that all 7 BioEnergetic Elements are flow triggers. Without the Thrive State, it is difficult for flow to exist. Perhaps, more definitively: With the Stress/Survival State, flow is nearly impossible.

When asked about his experience on the Diamond Princess a year after the Yokohama quarantine, Captain Gennaro Arma of the cruise line said,

---

204   "Neuroscience Based Training to Help You Accomplish More, in Less Time, with Greater Ease," Flow Research Collective, www.flowresearchcollective.com/training.

"A diamond is a chunk of coal that did well under pressure. I would like to think we'll be remembered as one big family that, under some very challenging times, remained united with sacrifice and went through these problems." Although diamonds aren't actually made from coal (they are made from carbon deposits which are more insignificant than coal itself), Captain Arma did remind us of the three necessary ingredients to turn these insignificant carbon deposits into diamonds: heat, pressure, and time. And once formed, that diamond is nearly indestructible. I've found that these three ingredients are almost the universal law to create anything great in life—the human body, great works of art, extraordinary companies, and every audacious human accomplishment.

I helped many individuals and organizations achieve the Thrive State. What I can say is that the strategy for every organization is different—customized for size, work environments, workflows, and current state. Still, the blueprint for achieving human potential is identical—the commitment to make and act upon the choices that will evolve us into the best versions of ourselves for service to others.

5 to Thrive

1. Just like the human body is an ecosystem made up of individual cells, families, teams, and organizations are ecosystems made up of individuals.

2. Ecosystems share 3 common traits: independence, interdependence, and state dependence all of which need to be optimized for the ecosystem as a whole to function at its best.

3. Cultivating the state of an ecosystem begins with each individual and can spread throughout the system through mirror neurons and other biological receptors.

4. The Thrive State Advantage: Organizations that are in the Thrive State are more productive, engaged, and prosperous.

5. The Thrive State activates more flow—optimal state of consciousness which allows us to feel our best and perform our best.

CHAPTER 12

CREATING LASTING IMPACT

By now you should be aware that the Thrive State is an energetic state of being and consciousness that activates the biology of optimal health, longevity, and peak performance and optimizes our human potential. It is the most authentic expression of YOU. It is the YOU in your natural state. In organizations, the Thrive State, is what creates better performance, productivity, and prosperity.

That being the case, why aren't more people in the Thrive State? Why do we find so many people (and organizations) falling short of their true potential?

I want you to remember the word IMPACT. Remember: Our choices and subsequent actions create the state of our bodies and environment. IMPACT is the simple framework that allows us to take actions consistently towards the Thrive State—to become the best versions of ourselves. Let me briefly introduce the IMPACT framework here:

I'M = Know your "I Am," who you want to become. Have a vision for your identity and the life you want to live.

P = Pause and create space

A = Awareness

C = Choice

T = Take action

This framework has allowed many individuals and organizations to unlock a new level of health, performance, and vitality within themselves to create sustained happiness, success, and prosperity for themselves and the people they serve. I am confident you will receive similar results if you apply this framework into your own life. In the following pages, I will unpack why people make choices that undermine their potential, and reveal how the IMPACT framework is the key to reaching and staying in the Thrive State.

To understand why we make choices that may sabotage our potential, let's revisit "old neuronal wiring" which I reference In Chapter 8: Mindset is Everything. Scientists are beginning to understand more about a part of the brain called the Default Mode Network (DMN).[205,206] This is one of the most primitive parts of the brain, which starts developing in utero. Neuroscientists have mapped out the relevant area of the brain, which includes the medial prefrontal cortex; the posterior cingulate cortex; the hippocampus (our memory center); and the amygdala (our fear center), as well as parts of the inferior parietal lobe.

The DMN is the brain's autopilot mode whose function is to keep us safe and help us survive. From an early age, the DMN functions like a great big sponge, soaking up massive amounts of information concerning just about everything we encounter—from our interactions with those closest to us such as parents, siblings, relatives, teachers, and friends—to experiences

205 Smallwood, Jonathan et al. "The default mode network in cognition: a topographical perspective." *Nature reviews. Neuroscience* vol. 22,8 (2021): 503-513.

206 Smallwood, Jonathan et al. "The neural correlates of ongoing conscious thought." *iScience* vol. 24,3 102132. 1 Feb. 2021.

within our wider community and society, much of which we receive from television and media. Whether for good or for bad, these inputs shape our models and beliefs about the world and where we fit in. Because its function is to help us survive, the DMN is constantly looking for what can hurt us.

Due to the link between the amygdala (fear) and hippocampus (memory), the DMN remembers our fears and traumas—particularly the most emotionally charged experiences. Why? To prevent us from being hurt again in the future. Because the DMN is continually protecting us from harm, it holds a negativity bias. That is, it pays more attention to perceived negative experiences. This is the source of the Automatic Negative Thoughts (ANTS) that Dr. Daniel Amen, MD discusses in his book, *Change Your Brian, Change Your Life*. This is where our limiting beliefs and disempowering stories live—beliefs like "I'm not good enough" or "I'm not worthy of love."

The DMN is generally programmed in early childhood, and it is the default operating system that runs in the background when we are not paying attention; hence the "auto-pilot" aspect. Its patterns and networks are programmed largely before our higher brain centers have a chance to develop. The speed of the DMN's synaptic firing is usually much faster than that coming from the conscious brain centers. For example, if you touch a hot stove, you quickly pull away. From a very early age, your brain and nervous system have learned and associated high heat with harm and pain. These deeply rooted neural networks allow your arm to reflexively pull back to protect you. This automatic, unconscious, and extremely reactive trait has obvious evolutionary survival advantages. Imagine if you had to consciously sense the heat from the stove, and then consciously be aware to fire the neurons to move your arm. The additional time and processing power of your nervous system might have caused your arm to turn into burnt toast.

Our early childhood brains develop models and beliefs about the world. Just like the way we pull our hands back from a hot stove without conscious thought, we have adaptive thoughts, beliefs, feelings, and behaviors we develop at an early age that keep us safe. This is why so many neuroscientists call the DMN the seat of the ego. These adaptive mechanisms may include:

- The need to fit in, because to be outed by a tribe is dangerous.
- The need to please people, because others' approval is what allows us to stay in the tribe.
- The need to achieve external success, because success is necessary to be worthy and to receive love.

We know the children of alcoholic parents tend to be either meek and subservient in order to avoid belligerent behavior, or exemplify rage and anger to challenge the alcoholic parent. These coping mechanisms can affect interactions with siblings or peers.[207] Aggressive behavior typically follows these children as they get older and if left untreated, increases the risk for physical and mental illness, unemployment, poverty, and/or criminal behavior.[208] The irrational pre-programmed fear and belief that we are not good enough or even adequate tells us we aren't worthy of an essential nutrient for survival... LOVE.

Conversely, parents who are fully, or even partially aware of the DMN's impact on their own behaviors and how that affects their child's development can make conscious choices with their words and behaviors to minimize their child's fear and negativity. Because I now have a solid understanding of how my DMN affected me, I am more cognizant of how I interact with my daughter and bonus-daughter. Certainly, I can't control outside influences (e.g., schoolmates, friends), but I can act as a counter-balance, offering positivity, support, and love.

Although the DMN has some evolutionary advantages, if we are not aware of it—and most people are not aware—we make choices from this unconscious, autopilot, survival mode of the brain. From what operating system

---

207   Edwards, Ellen P et al. "The development of aggression in 18 to 48 month old children of alcoholic parents." *Journal of abnormal child psychology* vol. 34,3 (2006): 409-23.

208   Scott, James G et al. "The aggressive child." *Journal of paediatrics and child health* vol. 54,10 (2018): 1165-1169.

do you think choices were made that led to war in Ukraine, the attack on the U.S. capitol, or George Floyd's death and the subsequent riots? We also are fighting a virus impacting the entire globe that some people labeled the "China virus." To date, that terminology has precipitated nearly 4,000 anti-Asian hate crimes. What operating system do you think is at work in those situations? All of this reminds me of my childhood, when my DMN was programmed. As I discussed in Chapter 1, the stressful events of early childhood heavily impacted my "old programming," and I lived my early life trying to satisfy my need to feel worthy.

The DMN is the self-critic. It's the part of us that gets anxious about the past, or worries about the future. That is our Ego. The spiritual biologist Bruce Lipton, PhD asserts that the movie "The Matrix" is more than a movie, it's a documentary. You may recall in the movie that humans experience their reality through a series of computer programs that are plugged into their nervous system. These humans can't tell the difference between these programs and true reality, so they base their decisions on these programs rather than free will. A similar analogy is the fish in water. Do the fish realize they are in water or are they oblivious to it? The DMN is our matrix. It is the water we swim in.

You may be wondering how living in the DMN leads to disease and poor performance. Let's use the bioenergetic model and the choices I made to reprogram my brain. First and foremost, MENTAL choices held me back. My old programming defined me as: "I'm not enough," "I need success to be worthy of love." I sought success by putting myself first, instead of lifting others. Second, I made poor SPIRITUAL choices. I wore the mask of not connecting. When I put on my white coat, I chose to interact through that, instead of making a deep connection and sharing my authentic self. Third, poor SOCIAL choices. I participated superficially in social settings, without genuine emotion; I was socially disengaged. Fourth, untamed EMOTIONAL choices. Stress, anxiety, worry and fear led me to daily habits which did nothing other than make my health suffer. Fifth, poor PHYSICAL choices. I failed to prioritize sleep, ate unhealthily, and put off exercising. All my choices created a bioenergetic state—one that wasn't good. I had immersed myself in the Stress/Survival State, which ultimately led to inflammation and chronic disease. My choices were made from the DMN (based on survival and fear), and it's clear how easily they activated the Stress State in my body.

You may recall that my dying patient Ishmael gave me the opening to begin making new choices. New experiences gave me a new outlook on life. I started to sleep, eat, and move better. By making better PHYSICAL choices, I started to optimize my biochemistry and hormones. Guess what? I started to feel better. I had more energy, and I felt alive. I experienced an improved EMOTIONAL state and made choices from that place. Because I felt better, I connected better with my community and tribe. This led to positive SOCIAL choices. I wanted to share my happiness and all I had learned about health for the purpose of empowering others. Armed with better SPIRITUAL choices, I began believing everything happens *for* me, and not *to* me. I came to understand that my choices create my health, and my reality. I started recognizing that my story—my biography—dictates my biology. I could now make better MENTAL choices. As I started to master the art of living by making more conscious choices in these bioenergetic elements, I began to live in the Thrive State. By combining this with anti-aging and regenerative medicine and biohacking technologies, I've been able to reverse my diabetes and high blood pressure, lose inflammatory visceral fat, and biologically age backwards.

In the book the *Blue Zones*, author Dan Buettner identified five regions of the world with the highest concentration of centenarians: Sardinia, Italy; Okinawa, Japan; Icaria, Greece; Nicoya Peninsula, Costa Rica; and Loma Linda, California. Dan and his research team of researchers identified common traits as to why they lived so long.[209] As it turns out, these traits are nearly identical to the bioenergetic elements I discuss in this book. The Blue Zone inhabitants didn't intentionally seek to become the longest-lived

---

209 Buettner, Dan, and Sam Skemp. "Blue Zones: Lessons From the World's Longest Lived." *American journal of lifestyle medicine* vol. 10,5 318-321. 7 Jul. 2016.

people on the planet. Rather, that was a byproduct of *how* they chose to live, and more importantly, *who* they chose to be.

Who do you choose to be? Who is the authentic you—the real you that lies beneath all the unconscious programming? It doesn't really matter if you're unable to remember or not, because you get to choose NOW. You don't need to have anything to be anything. You don't need to do anything to be anything. In other words, you don't need to be a billionaire to be wealthy. You don't need a job title to be confident. You don't need hundreds of Facebook friends to be a good friend. I used to think I needed all these external things to feel worthy, but it was just an illusion. I am worthy, and so are you.

You are whoever you say you are following these two simple words, "I AM..." Ask yourself: Who do you desire to be? Do you want to be happy, joyous, playful, confident, courageous, integrous, generous, playful, successful, blissful, or grateful? This is yours to choose. No job title, amount in your bank account, things you possess, or number of friends ever defines who you are. You define yourself. That's it. You choose. Your task is to place a flag in the sand, create your identity, and have a bold vision of your life. Let your flag stand strong, unapologetic in the breeze, the wind, or the gale. This is where you make your choices from.

Yet, if your flag is ever at risk of falling down... if that old programming resurfaces, I want you to PAUSE (create space) and ACT (have Awareness, Choose, Take action). Every time you have that unhealthy food craving, or feel lazy on the couch, or are triggered by your spouse... create space. Go for a walk, sit in a garden or park, do breathwork or a meditation, or simply take 10 deep breaths in through your nose and out through your mouth. Focus on a longer 8 to 10 second exhalation. When you do this, you activate your parasympathetic nervous system, which then allows the space for you to ACT.

It is essential to have Awareness of your trigger(s). Do you feel triggered because of old programming? Is it that old story of "I'm not worthy"? Or that belief that being overweight is in your genes? Perhaps your spouse or co-worker triggered this old wound of "not being good enough." It is equally essential to be aware of the thoughts and the emotions that this specific trigger elicited within your body. Where is your body feeling these emotional sensations? Is there a physicality, or a symptom, to the sensations? You recognize the unconscious patterns at work when you are able to identify and label these sensations within your body.

I've learned to be grateful that I am able to recognize these uncomfortable feelings and thoughts. They provide cues as to the parts of my unconscious I can—and should—work on. So, be curious as to why these feelings come up. Can you remember a moment in your past when you experienced something familiar? What naive thought or belief might you have interpreted about yourself when you felt that way? The more you practice this step of Awareness, the more you realize the unconscious programs that your mind has buried away. And when you start to see that programming as NOT YOU, just old programming, then you can really make a conscious choice.

Then Choose. Choose from that place of I AM that you identified previously. Who do you want to be? How do you want to show up? What choice is aligned with your Thrive State? Listen to your ideal inner voice. Is it kind, nurturing, joyous, and loving?

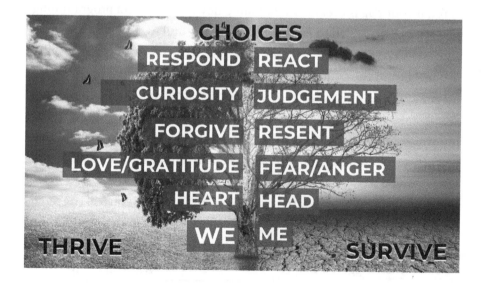

Once you make that new choice, you immediately Take action. If you chose to be loving and connected in the face of an argument with your spouse, then maybe your action looks something like saying, "Oh honey, I'm sorry I reacted. I didn't mean that. I just got triggered by some old programming. I want us to be connected. Can we start over in a few minutes?" (I've used this one a lot.) Perhaps, you accompany this with a light touch on your spouse's arm (physical action), or you gently take his/her hand.

Make the conscious choice of acceptance over judgment; forgiveness rather than resentment; service instead of taking. Every time you make this new choice, you are rewiring your entire body and nervous system into the Thrive State, and you are upgrading your operating system from the non-functional, old programming.

Certainly, old programming will come up from time to time. However, the level, amplitude, and intensity of your attention, your consciousness, and your conviction to your I AM vision are what gives you the power to override the DMN Programming.

As a mnemonic from this process, remember the word IMPACT.

Know your **I AM** = the vision and choice of your identity
and the life you want to live

P = Pause and create space

A = Awareness

C = Choice

T = Take action

Think for a moment on how the world could change if more people used this IMPACT framework. Imagine how the positive conscious choices could elevate the individual and collective state in which we live. What would it look and feel like if more and more of us were in the Thrive State?

By elevating our own personal state—our individual vibration—we change our individual biology, and that energy permeates outwards and impacts others. Your children... my children... the planet will experience this new vibration, this new programming. You and I become the seed of a new Blue Zone. So, make the choice you want to see in the world and choose to create a beautiful masterpiece of a life. That's the art of living, and it's the best medicine you can provide for yourself and humanity.

5 to Thrive

1. The state of our bodies (and organizations) is the result of our collective choices and subsequent actions.

2. The Default Mode Network (DMN) is a primitive operating system that is programmed through our childhood experiences which some scientists consider to be the seat of the ego.

3. The negativity and survival bias of the DMN creates the self-critic, disempowering stories, and limiting beliefs in our subconscious.

4. Unconscious choices made through the adaptive programming of the DMN sabotages our health and progress in life, relationships, and business.

5. The IMPACT framework is a methodology for making conscious choices towards the Thrive State and becoming the best versions of ourselves.

YOU ARE YOUR BEST MEDICINE

As I write this Conclusion, we are starting to come out of the global COVID-19 pandemic. Life will likely never be the same as it was pre-pandemic. In the last chapter, I've mentioned the three necessary ingredients to create greatness: pressure, heat, and time. In the past few years, people have dealt with so much pressure. And not only have people endured, but they were able to bring the heat with their persistent pursuit of their passion and purpose. In this setting of pressure and heat, the past few years and the time ahead will only act as the incubator for the seeds of greatness to emerge.

When I was writing the first edition of this book, the idea of "thriving" seemed out of reach; so many people were simply surviving, and unfortunately, some didn't. Over the past few years, all of our BioEnergetic Elements were likely in disarray: we couldn't go to our gyms; shopping for food was a logistical nightmare; our sleep was shot; we couldn't physically socialize with our friends and family without constant fear of infection; and our stress levels were through the roof.

I certainly remembered what that felt like. I felt it myself, so much so that I have even had moments of "imposter syndrome." I remember sitting at my desk, staring out the window that overlooked a yard full of dead grass, and thinking to myself, *Yeah, I'm an authority on thriving.*

A year before the COVID lockdowns in Los Angeles, I had sold the fancy, ornate house that my years in the medical grind had paid for. It was the last break with the old me, the one that had prioritized the appearance of success over genuine happiness. The house I had moved into was smaller and less private. And right around the move, COVID became a global pandemic. My partner Tiffany's industry shut down during the quarantine, and I saw my savings and investments take a very big hit. Stress and anxiety were in the air, and in my head.

In my former home, I would find myself staring out through a set of beautifully ornate, massive glass windows, with panoramic views of the Silver Lake Reservoir, the Griffith Observatory, and the Hollywood sign. The view I currently had to look forward to, I knew, was a neglected front porch in a neighborhood I didn't love, bookended by a liquor store on each corner of my block. The tranquility of my former quiet environment, with the smell of well-kept shrubbery and flowers, would be replaced with the scents and sounds of the inner city, replete with car-honking and day-old takeout.

I wasn't just nervous for myself; I was nervous for my new family. Tiffany and I had just learned we were pregnant, and so we had decided to move in together—along with Tiffany's beautiful six-year-old daughter, Kira. This was the first home we would be sharing together as a family. I wanted it to be perfect, but it didn't feel that way.

But, as if it were magic, Kira took to the new home immediately. When we arrived, she ran to her "new" bedroom to jump on her "new" bed (in reality, a hand-me-down). Next was her joy over the front porch—she excitedly exclaimed that she had never had a porch before, seemingly oblivious to the fact that my yard space had shrunk. She was overjoyed, running circles of excitement in her euphoric six-year-old state of mind. And not a day has passed since that she isn't just as excited and grateful for her new home.

There's nothing better than a child at play. Children are completely in the present moment. And when they feel joy, that joy is untinged by irony, or jealousy, or self-doubt. Children at play feel the pull of joy. When we are able to feel that pure form of joy, whether as children or adults, we are our truest selves.

Even as the author of Thrive State, I admit that the thoughts, feelings, and reactions of my Default Mode network—the unworthiness, the not enoughness—still come up. I don't think these thoughts will ever fully go away. However with practice, I can be more aware of the constant chattering of the DMN, and apply the IMPACT framework to recenter myself. But every now and then, I'll take those gentle life reminders and lessons from my children. Kira's joyful reaction to our home blasted me out of my imposter syndrome, reminding me of the power of mindset.

A single change in our perspective, in the story we tell ourselves, allows us to see our authentic selves and shift our minds and bodies from a Stress State to a Thrive State of being. And when we are our authentic selves, there is no imposter syndrome.

There was another moment of pressure involving my other daughter during the pandemic. I wasn't able to attend any of Tiffany's prenatal visits as her pregnancy progressed. Forty weeks in, her OB suggested we induce. It was January 2021, and our hospital had just started letting dads back into the maternity ward. I was about to be a first time (biological) dad, and I arrived at the hospital excited, taking selfies and documenting everything. A nurse began an IV on Tiffany to begin the induction process, then said to me, "Dr. Vuu, it'll be a few hours before anything happens. Get some rest."

I lay down in the hard hospital bed and begin to fall asleep. About 30 minutes later, I heard two footsteps. I didn't think anything of it, but then, I heard four. Then a team of people rushed into the room with an ultrasound machine. Part of me was thinking, am I dreaming? The doctor put the ultrasound on my fiancé Tiffany, then turned to me: "Dr Vuu, your baby might die if we don't have an emergency C-section right now.

We had to make a difficult choice, and we ended up in the operating room. When I first heard the baby cry, I thought, "Thank God." They asked me if I wanted to cut the cord. I cut the cord and then I realized something was wrong. She wasn't moving much, and alarms started beeping. I looked at her oxygen saturation levels. They were dropping: 95 down to 90 to 85 to

80. As I looked around, the same people who were congratulating me just moments ago wouldn't look me in the eye. Then I felt this hand on my shoulder. "Dr Vuu, we need to take her to the NICU now."

Moments later our OB said, "Dr Vuu, she was born with her cord wrapped around her neck and ankle." WHAT?!?! My mind filled with worry: Was she deprived of oxygen? How long was it there? Will she have brain damage? Will she have the choice to live? My newborn daughter didn't choose to have that cord wrapped around her neck. At that moment, I didn't know if she'd be able to make any choices. In that moment, I was deeply reminded about the gift and the power of our choices—EVEN in the darkest of times—to find the deeper meaning, to access our hidden resources, and to become the best versions of ourselves.

This was a moment of pressure I've never experienced before. I remember thinking "Why is this happening to me?" I wanted to blame the doctors. I wanted to blame the hospital. Then I employed my IMPACT framework.

I Paused and created space. Then I took 10 deep breaths. I had the Awareness that I was reacting, not responding. I Chose—I chose the belief that everything happens for me, not to me. I Took action by asking different questions: How is this happening for me? Where's the gift at this moment?

Right when I asked that question, the nurse asked me if I wanted to hold my daughter for the first time. She had a tube down her nose, a tube down her mouth, and IVs in her arms. I thought, "Health complications or not, she is perfect just the way she is." Then my heart just cracked open, and I was reminded of how precious life is—how each of us who's been given this life is absolutely more than enough and worthy of love—even me. A huge wave of healing overcame me and washed away that old programming of "not enough" that had been lingering. It was happening *for* me, not to me. As I write this, Kaia Astara Vuu is a very happy and healthy two-year-old, which is another fantastic reason for me to be in the Thrive State.

Those were just a few examples of my own life where there was pressure. Each of us has our own versions of what pressure looked like. It is this pressure and time that reinforced this belief in me: WE choose our mindset, how we view the world, and how we react to change. In doing so, we choose our quality of life and, ultimately, our health and performance. You and your choices are the most powerful medicine any doctor can prescribe.

My life has taught me that each and every one of us must discover ourselves—and then trust ourselves. As we journey through life, seeking a higher consciousness and understanding of the world in which we live is a choice, one that benefits us as well as the people around us. Some may call this *wisdom* or *enlightenment*. I call it the Thrive State. Deliberate choices and corresponding actions in all facets of life—from the physiological to the psychological—allow us to thrive rather than simply react and survive. Live each day. Don't just survive each day to make it to the next.

Self-discovery is a highly personal process, of course. Your life choices are different from my life choices—or, at least, they should be—and there is no one "correct" way to live your life. Bundled up with all of this is the notion of authenticity. There are a lot of definitions for "authenticity," but let me propose a definition of my own: authenticity is a refusal to apologize for following your own bliss.

In my own journey, I have struggled with this. My authentic self is a comic, a creative, a storyteller. I spent evenings as a kid entertaining myself in front of the mirror in my family's cramped apartment in Los Angeles's Chinatown. I would spend hours making up stories, trying out outrageous accents, and practicing jokes. When I could coax a laugh out of someone, I felt joy—even if that laugh was accompanied by an eye roll or a muttering of, "You're so corny, Kien." My class-clown personality was something I was born with; it was an energy that I brought with me into every interaction. It was authentically me.

But I often didn't feel I had the space to explore this part of myself. Like many other immigrant parents, my mother and father made it clear to me—from a very early age—that I was expected to get a job that would put me on firm financial and societal footing. My dreams of comedy or acting definitely did not fit that description.

My experience training to be a doctor—from medical school to residency—isolated that part of my personality even further. Medical school is *Serious*, with a capital "S." Every decision you make is imbued with a sense of gravitas. Light-heartedness is seen as a poor fit for a doctor, and joking is discouraged. I remember several times when my mentors would tell me, "You need to calm down," or "Try not to be so animated." It was difficult advice to receive. These were people I looked up to, my role models. But at the same time, their feedback sat uncomfortably with me. I felt that I was being asked to repress a significant part of myself.

My mentors all wanted me to succeed—but they themselves had been trained to see "success" through the lens of professional accomplishment. They were comparing me to the medical field's vision of the ideal doctor: solemn, focused, and maybe even a little robotic. I was told I had to act a certain way in order to succeed as a physician, but this ideal of success allowed very little room for authenticity—and so, at my core, I always instinctively rejected it.

Now, here's how I know that cracking jokes is a part of my authentic personality: because even when my superiors told me to "turn off" that side of myself, I couldn't. It was too deeply ingrained within me. I was the resident who would show up to work wearing bow ties and glitter pants. I was the one who would liven up a slow shift at the hospital by prank calling my friends and colleagues stationed on other wards—requesting obviously made-up procedures and coming up with crazy medical scenarios at three o'clock in the morning. And I won't lie. Some people thought I was a little too loud, a little too much. But others told me that they appreciated how I was bringing joy and personality into the hospital, especially during the hardest days—the days when our team lost a patient, or when we were nearing the end of another brutally long and non-stop shift.

And most importantly, I could see the effect that my light was having on many of my patients. In their laughs and smiles, I could feel them responding to me. It wasn't even that they found my jokes to be funny—I mean, if I'm being honest, some of my jokes are downright corny. But they were reacting to the presence of my authenticity. I was authentically there in the room with them. I was not hiding anything about who I was. I was more than just "the doctor." I was a real person, standing by their side as they battled through major health scares and even life-and-death scenarios.

I have sat with patients for whom their trips to the hospital had become a source of increasing pain. Maybe it was because their prognosis was poor, or because their disease was progressing, or because they were not responding well to the treatment. And I have had these patients tell me that they found my personality—my light-hearted manner, my quirks, my jokes—to be a source of healing and joy. Even amidst the frustrations and pain and uncertainty of their hospital visit, it gave them something to look forward to.

It is truly an honor to offer that little source of healing to my patients who need it. And it just wouldn't be possible if I wasn't being authentic with them. If I was hiding who I was, it would be impossible for my patients to feel that sense of connection with me. There is no "ideal doctor" who can offer them that sense of connection. There's only me. The one-and-only, authentic me. Glitter pants and all.

I hope that I can encourage you to do the same. There is a lot of strength to be gained from being your authentic self. Only when you are truly, authentically you can you truly thrive. Here are a few of my recommendations for how to thrive—physically, mentally, emotionally, and spiritually—by fortifying your own authenticity.

Trust your body, your instincts, and your inner desires. Your intuition (i.e., "gut instinct") is encoded in your genetic makeup. Don't live in a construct that doesn't fit you. Of course, you must *know thyself* first, to know whether any such constructs are out of line with your true self or not. Choose your path, follow your instincts, trust your inner being, and your trajectory will be in the direction of the Thrive State.

Release your authentic self and live fully engaged with the world around you. This is the heat we bring into the equation of Greatness = Pressure + Heat + Time. This is who we are authentically. If we bring our persistent passion and purpose to life, we bring the heat.

Once you are able to trust your inner being, free yourself from that which has held you physically or mentally captive. Optimize your BioEnergetic Enhancers to break free from the chronic disease that may have limited you from full self-expression or active participation within relationships and social or community engagement. Once you are unencumbered by the cages that limit your potential, work towards rediscovering your purpose, finding happiness, and then share it with the world. Remember: we are in our most natural and most joyous state when we can *know* who we are, and when we *express* who we are to others.

Follow the Feel-Good Rule. If you are questioning whether a specific action or encounter will bring you to your Thrive State, ask yourself: *How does this food/activity/person feel one hour from now, one day from now, one week from now, and one month from now?* If it's positive all the way through, you're on to something. If not, reconsider.

My intention is for this book to be a blueprint by which readers can gain inspiration, self-discovery, and guidance for improving health and well-being. I created it to be an overview of the many areas of health (physical, mental, emotional, spiritual) so as to maximize the various energies surrounding us. Now that you have read this book, think about your personal goals and select one or two areas to focus on (to start), whether it's getting better sleep, or starting an exercise program, or eating better. Whatever your goal(s) may be, go back and reread the relevant chapter and implement some of the ideas I presented. (I've also created a cheat sheet on the following page to remind you of the bioenergetic enhancers you'll want to incorporate into your life).

Each of the 7 BioEnergetic Elements has its own unique power to improve your healthspan and performance, and as you master one, you will feel its positive, energizing influence in your life. The 7 Elements build upon one another, so tackle another, and another. Remember, every new habit implemented creates energetic momentum to make it easier to tackle new habits and to get you into the Thrive State. And if you crave more knowledge on any specific topic, I encourage you to seek it—either from the resources I noted, or from people in your personal social community, or from the Internet (the worldwide social community) from experts you trust. I've also included some additional resources at thrivestatebook.com/resources. Learning should never cease.

For many, seeking optimal health and performance (human potential) is part of their DNA, so why not utilize our knowledge of epigenetics? We know that genetics do not determine our health destiny... and thank goodness. If you happen to have a family history of heart disease, cancer, type 2 diabetes, or another chronic disease, remind yourself—often, if necessary—you can choose not to have that disease. Genetic predisposition does not equal genetic predetermination. Your genes interact with your environment (sleep, nutrition, movement, stress, mindset, relationships, and purpose) to create who you are at any given moment in time. By making positive environmental choices, your good genes will be turned on; your bad genes will remain turned off; your telomeres will remain lengthy; your gut microbiome will remain in homeostasis; and your immune system will function appropriately and robustly. You have the power to offset your risk of suffering some of the most horrible diseases, such as Alzheimer's. If you currently have a chronic disease (like I once did), make a conscious commitment to health and back it up with deliberate action to activate your body's innate healing ability. On the other side of your conscious efforts is abundant health, longevity, and optimal performance. My friends, I don't know whether you realize it or not, but just by living through these past few years, you are forging the diamond of greatness that is your life. Trust yourself, empower yourself, and you will thrive. YOU are your best medicine!

	BioEnergetic Enhancers	BioEnergetic Detractors
SLEEP	• Regular exercise • Good nutrition • Early-morning sunshine • Stress management • Nighttime before bed routine • Blackout lights • Chilled room	• Late-day stimulants (caffeine, nicotine) • Some prescription drugs, including sleep medications • Illicit drugs • Stress, worry • Blue light
NUTRITION	• Organic, minimally processed • Sustainably raised meat • Clean drinking water • Good fats • Intermittent fasting	• Pesticides and other toxins • Factory-farmed meat • Polluted drinking water • Sugar, processed foods, bad oils
MOVEMENT	• Daily activity • Structured exercise	• Inactivity • Prolonged sitting
STRESS/ EMOTIONS	• Regular stress management (Yoga, qigong, massage, laughter yoga, exercise, sex) • Being in nature • Professional therapy • Cultivating emotional intelligence	• Internalization • Social isolation • Self-medicating with drugs • Lack of awareness of negative emotions • Reacting to negative emotions

	BioEnergetic Enhancers	BioEnergetic Detractors
MINDSET	• An open mind, sense of curiosity, willingness to learn • Regular social engagement • Forgiveness • Awareness and ability to shift disempowering beliefs	• A closed mind with narrow focus • Social isolation • Resentment, anger • Believing your negative self-talk
RELATIONSHIPS & COMMUNITY	• Positive relationships • Social engagement	• Toxic relationships • Social isolation
PURPOSE	• Eudaimonic happiness (primarily) • Self-awareness & self-acceptance • Selfless (being a "giver") • Gratitude and joy • You lt	• Hedonic happiness (solely) • Lack of self-awareness & self-acceptance • Selfishness (being a "taker")

STRENGTHENING YOUR PATH FORWARD

While I am confident that anyone who has thoroughly read this book has received the foundational knowledge, skills, and motivation for optimizing their BioEnergetic State, there is always room for improvement. As you may recall in the preface, there are two main approaches in the human performance and longevity space. By far, the most empowering are the concepts of epigenetics and YOU being your best medicine. The choices that we make dictate our biology. This is what I've termed the "Art of Living." Then, of course, there is the blossoming and exponential growth of medical advances and technology which promises to push the human lifespan further than what we thought possible—to which I call the "Science of Longevity."

In this section, I will briefly highlight some of the technologies in the longevity space that are offered in longevity practices across the country, including my own concierge practice and business consulting firm. My work is centered around elevating human and organizational performance and longevity.

A proven formula which I've used both in my concierge practice and shared in my Thrive State Accelerator program (kienvuu.com/accelerator), is what I call the HERO Prescription (Rx).

This methodology focuses on enhancing one's quality of life and overall vibrancy through assessing and restoring an individual's (or organization's) BioEnergetic State, then utilizing modern science to upgrade the intricate inner balance of nutrition, hormones, and optimization of cellular bioenergetics. The HERO Rx consists of 4 categories.

- **Hunger:** Hunger is the engine of self-optimization. Know your compelling WHY. What drives you to succeed? Why is change a must for you? Using the HERO Rx, my clients and I spend a lot of time examining their motivations and rediscovering what truly propels them to change.
- **Energy:** This category is all about the BioEnergetic Model, bringing the clients into a more optimized state at the cellular level—something you now know as the Thrive State.
- **Reclamation:** Reclamation is about defining your identity; rediscovering all the discarded joys, passions, and interests that made you who you are but that life's many demands have supplanted. Ultimately, it is your authentic sense of self, your true greatness, that will drive you to solidify the changes into habits that will keep you in the Thrive State.
- **Optimization:** Drawing from time-tested wisdom, traditions and modern science, I work with my clients to optimize their health and performance, keeping each of them at the top of their mental, physical, and emotional game.

The Hunger, Energy, and Reclamation components are really the Art of Living components of getting into the Thrive State, while the Optimization component is the Science of Longevity. After working with hundreds of high performing individuals, I can say that spending money on the Optimization component of the HERO Rx without focusing on the other three components first is generally a waste of an investment. Why? Because you want to use the science of longevity to elevate the optimized state from your art of living, and not use it to make up for the poor state created from your choices.

Through the execution of this HERO Rx, I have consistently seen individuals experience increased energy and vitality, optimized weight, enhanced mental, physical, and emotional performance, improved mood, satisfying sexual experiences, and quality sleep.

So, before any of the Optimization work begins, I recommend a thorough assessment of the individual's current BioEnergetic elements and lifestyle choices.

Advances in Diagnostic Testing

In the Science of Longevity realm, I deeply believe in advanced anatomical and functional testing to assess the physical state of the body.

We first perform a comprehensive laboratory analysis that includes a complete metabolic panel, complete blood cell count, NMR lipid panel, complete hormone panel, and specific nutrients. Additionally, depending on client history, symptoms, or concerns, environmental toxins testing, indolent infections, and micronutrient profiles can also be performed. Because "leaky gut" is so pervasive today and often a contributing cause of chronic disease, microbiome analysis and gut pathogen identification are paramount to evaluating the health of the G.I. tract and its impact on immune, brain, and skin health. Each program takes in account the individual's health and performance goals, and clients receive a customized lifestyle plan to optimize these areas. I'm also a fan of more advanced testing in the longevity space which include the following:

Full Body MRI utilizes magnetic resonance imaging (MRI) technology in the capacity of early detection, rather than symptom evaluation and late-stage diagnosis. Prenuvo (prenuvo.com) scans can check for upwards of 350+ different conditions, including brain aneurysms and cancerous tumors in their early stages. Early detection benefits patients by saving lives—faster, more frequent monitoring and treatment for better outcomes.

TruDiagnostic Epigenetic Testing is a new diagnostic tool which is sure to change every area of medicine where age is a risk factor for chronic disease. TruDiagnostic (trudiagnostic.com) is a leader in the field of epigenetic analysis. Using a single drop of blood, it is possible to determine the body's biological age, the pace of aging, the immune system's aging trajectory, and even predict how the human face might age.

Galleri Multi-Cancer Early Detection Test detects 50+ different types of cancer, most of which do not have routine or recommended screenings. The Galleri Test (galleri.com) uses DNA obtained from a blood draw to detect methylation patterns, which may indicate the presence of cancer. With high accuracy, this "liquid biopsy" predicts the cancer's origin. This test does not detect specific genetic mutations, nor does it predict a person's risk for developing cancer.

GlycanAge is a biological age test that is used to compare with one's chronological age. It can also be a good indicator of the effects of lifestyle improvements, such as nutrition, exercise, stress, etc. Using GlycanAge (glycanage.com) over time can assess the aging or anti-aging effects of major life events, in addition to lifestyle modification, on health and well-being.

Biohacking Tools for Performance and Longevity

Dave Asprey, known to many as the Father of Biohacking, defines biohacking as "the art and science of changing the environment around you and inside you, so you have more control over your own biology. It's what you put in your mouth, it's the air you breathe, it's the light you're exposed to. Most people have twice as much energy potential, but they're doing hundreds of small things that hold them back."

Biohacking includes both the lifestyle choices and the technologies that we can implement to both detect and change our biology. There are numerous ways to incorporate methods of biohacking your body and mind into your daily routine. While this entire book is really the lifestyle "biohacks" to get you into the Thrive State, here are some technologies I enjoy:

Ice Bath is used following an athletic event or intense training session as a form of recovery. Immersing the entire body for 10 - 15 minutes at 50 - 59°F decreases core temperature; constricts blood vessels; and slows down blow flow throughout the body. Benefits include providing relief from sore or aching muscles; limiting inflammation for quicker recovery; decreasing the effects of heat and humidity; training the vagus nerve to handle stress better; and improving sleep.

Red Light Therapy (RLT) is a treatment that exposes various parts of the body to low levels of red or near-infrared light with a lamp, device, or laser. Mitochondria within cells exposed to the light absorb the heat energy and in turn, generate more energy themselves. The theory behind the use of RLT is that the cells will repair themselves, become healthier, and initiate healing in the applied areas. RLT is also called low-level laser therapy (LLLT), low-power laser therapy (LPLT), or photobiomodulation (PBM).

Infrared Sauna utilizes electromagnetic radiation to warm the body. Unlike a traditional sauna which heats the air, heat from infrared lamps penetrates the tissue directly. An advantage of infrared is that users can experience a more intense sweat at a lower temperature (120°F - 140°F vs. 150°F - 180°F) and achieve the same health benefits. Saunas are used to promote relaxation, better sleep, relief from sore joints and muscles, detoxification, better skin, weight loss, and improved circulation.

Pulsed Electromagnetic Field (PEMF) therapy employs soothing natural energy directed to specific body parts through a specialized magnetic device. PEMF stimulates cells and facilitates the body's ability for self-healing, self-regulation, and regeneration. PEMF also offers relief from muscle fatigue and pain after intense exercise or generalized chronic pain; reduces inflammation; supports relaxation; and increases energy levels.

These are just a few of the myriad biohacking tools available to improve performance, recovery, and longevity. My approach to biohacking is to occasionally try out a few tools on your own and see what works, and then build a stack of technologies that work best for you. To learn more about biohacking, you may want to attend one of a number of focused conferences, such as The Biohacking Conference (biohackingconference.com), The Health Optimisation Summit (summit.healthoptimisation.com), or the Biohacker Summit (new.biohackersummit.com). Additionally, I mention some of my other favorite biohacks in thrivestatebook.com/resources.

Medical Tools for Performance and Longevity

If aging—or anti-aging—is a concern, I offer clients hormone optimization and the latest in peptide and regenerative medicine. Peak performers seeking improved recovery time after exercise or optimal physical, mental, and/or sexual performance follow individually designed optimization protocols.

When it comes to optimizing our clients' BioEnergetic States (the "O" in "HERO"), we offer the following advanced therapies and treatments. (some of these treatments are still considered investigational at the time of this book's release):

- Peptide Therapy – This evolving area of medicine is utilized to treat age-related conditions (e.g., osteoporosis, muscle loss), inflammatory diseases, weight issues, sexual dysfunction, skin and hair problems, and much more. Naturally occurring peptides, or small proteins comprised of amino acids, are used as signaling molecules and hormones by the body. Peptide production fluctuates with age. Thus, synthetic peptides—administered as an injection, topical cream, orally, or nasally—have been used to restore biological pathways by imitating the function of naturally-occurring proteins that have decreased from previously optimal levels. Specific peptides utilized for performance attainment may include the following:

- Growth Hormone Secretagogues and Analogs: There are several small peptides that function to aid in the release or augment the effect of growth hormone on the body; a few of these compounds include Sermorelin, Ipamorelin, Hexarelin, and CJC1295, among others. These peptides upregulate growth hormone (GH) and IGF-1 levels in the body, leading to increased lean body mass; decreased body fat; improved sleep and bone density; reduced fatigue; improved memory and mood; and enhanced recovery.

- BPC-157: This protein is a derivative of Body Protection Compound (BPC), which occurs naturally in gastric juice and is known as the "healing molecule." BPC-157 is a shorter chain of 15 amino acids and helps reduce wound and tissue healing time, including G.I. tissue;

STRENGTHENING YOUR PATH FORWARD

stimulates new blood vessel growth; protects organs from toxic damage, particularly the liver; and protects neurons and other brain cells.

- **Semax:** This peptide quickly increases the expression of brain-derived neurotrophic factor (BDNF) and is used primarily as a nootropic, neuroprotectant, and immune system booster.

- **Selank:** This neuropeptide is the synthetic version of the body's own tuftsin, an immunostimulatory peptide. It is related to Semax in that it increases BDNF expression. Selank is most commonly used to treat anxiety, increase mental clarity, enhance memory and learning capacity, and improve mood.

- **PT141 (Bremelonotide):** Unlike other sexual-enhancement drugs, Bremelanotide PT-141 acts at the level of the brain, thus eliciting a natural sexual response. Melatonin ll (MT ll) is a peptide hormone that acts to increase sexual arousal by interacting with the hypothalamus in the brain. As a derivative of MT ll, Bremelanotide PT 141 induces sexual arousal by binding to melanocortin receptors in the hypothalamus. Studies suggest the effects of PT141 include heightened libido; improved symptoms of female sexual dysfunction; induction of erection in men suffering from erectile dysfunction; and improved sexual dysfunction on the level of the central nervous system. This peptide is one of the most popular peptides I prescribe for both men and women, for obvious reasons.

- **Thymosin Alpha 1:** This peptide is an immune booster. Made in the thymus, the gland responsible for generating our immune system, Thymosin Alpha 1 is prescribed to prevent viral, bacterial, and fungal infections. It does this by augmenting the function of your T cells, which are a major part of your adaptive immune system.

- **Thymosin Beta 4 (TB500):** TB500 is the tissue and muscle repair peptide and has been shown to be mainly involved in the healing of tissues. Found in almost all body tissues, it is released in response to trauma. It is a good option to use after surgery or an injury to skin, bone, cartilage, or tendons. It has also been shown to modulate tissue repair after a heart attack or any brain injury. It also has potent anti-inflammatory properties. Thymosin Beta 4 can also induce hair growth.

- Hormone Optimization – Hormone production within the body is key to optimal biological functioning, and both underproduction and overproduction can have deleterious effects. Sex hormones and growth hormones generally decrease with age, whereas stress hormones increase as a function of everyday stressors and poor coping mechanisms. Optimizing the body's hormones, whether through peptide therapy, hormone replacement, or behavioral modification, helps generate a state of homeostasis, allowing the body and mind to function more optimally.

- Nutrient Optimization – This is key to fueling the biological reactions within the human body and mind and, thus, avoiding disease and sub-optimal performance. Nutrient deficiencies can result from a variety of reasons, and these deficiencies can lead to poor cellular performance and chronic disease. Therefore, daily supplementation is generally recommended. As discussed in Chapter 5, a basic supplementation regimen should include vitamin D3, fish oil or Omega-3 fatty acids, magnesium, alpha-lipoic acid, CoQ10, and a high-quality multi-vitamin. Some of the supplements I personally take can be found at thrivestatebook.com/resources. At our clinics, we test for specific micronutrient deficiencies and develop a personalized supplementation plan to enhance the health, performance, and longevity goals of our clients.

- Gut Optimization – Maintaining a healthy, well-functioning G.I. tract is more important than previously thought. The composition of the microbiome—from the ratio of good to bad bacteria, to fungal overgrowth, to the presence of harmful parasites—is integral to immune, brain, and skin health. Maintaining the integrity of the gut lining keeps the pathogens, toxins, and undigested food proteins from entering the bloodstream and causing a massive inflammatory response from the immune system. A compromised gut barrier ("leaky gut") can be strengthened, and the microbiome can be balanced with optimized nutrition, stress reduction, and lifestyle modification. Specific digestive disorders, such as IBD, IBS, Crohn's disease, ulcerative colitis, and SIBO can also be addressed.

- **Intravenous Infusion Therapy** – IV therapy is not new but it is gaining popularity for its efficiency in delivering nutrients quickly for improved health, anti-aging properties, enhanced physical performance and endurance, and maximized brain power. Two very popular IV therapy options include:

- **Nutrient IV:** Various nutrient cocktails are created, which may include vitamins such as B3, methyl B12, B5, minerals (magnesium), and amino acids (acetyl-l-carnitine, glutamine, tryptophan, tyrosine, isoleucine, leucine, valine) in a quick (60 seconds or less) "push" or traditional drip infusion. Our proprietary formulas are designed to facilitate improved mood, better sleep, more intense workouts and quicker recovery, improved mental clarity, accelerated memory and mental acuity, and overall higher physical and mental performance.

- **NAD+ IV:** This infusion utilizes NAD+, a vitamin B3 derivative, which fuels the mitochondria—our cells' battery packs—to naturally increase mental and physical potential and to promote cellular repair and health. NAD+ is a vital coenzyme used to promote cellular repair, support cellular metabolism, and increase cellular energy. Because of these properties, proponents of NAD+ tout its physiological benefits to include increased energy, DNA protection and anti-aging effects, improved metabolism, adjunctive therapy for chronic disease, and potential to treat mental and neurological conditions. NAD+ IV can be used in combination with our nutrient IVs to assist individuals with anxiety, depression, PTSD, traumatic brain injury, neurological diseases, and problems with executive-level functioning. Unfortunately, the body's natural supply of NAD+ decreases with age, so replenishing NAD+ levels has been a valuable tool in the anti-aging and performance tool kit.

- **Regenerative Medicine** – Regenerative medicine is the field of science that aims to replace, heal, or "regenerate" human cells, tissues or organs to restore or establish normal function. Many of these technologies are still considered investigational, however, they are worth mentioning as they are the horizon of what's to come in the performance and longevity space.

- Platelet Rich Plasma (PRP) consists of two elements: plasma, or the liquid portion of blood, and platelets, a type of blood cell that plays an important role in healing throughout the body. Platelets are well-known for their clotting abilities, but they also contain growth factors that can trigger cell reproduction and stimulate tissue regeneration or healing in the treated area.

- Exosomes are packets of cellular information that contain a variety of healing messenger molecules including growth factors, mRNA, microRNA, DNA, and lipids. They are mediators of near and long-distance intercellular communication in health and disease and affect various aspects of cell biology.

- Stem cells are special human cells that are able to develop into many different cell types. This can range from muscle cells to brain cells. In some cases, they can also fix damaged tissues.

These regenerative biologic products have been used in a variety ways, including healing injured tissue (from trauma, surgery, stroke, heart attacks, degenerative disease, and more), regrowing hair, improving sexual function, enhancing general well-being and longevity, and others. While still investigational, these technologies along with organ regeneration—the process of implanting or integrating man-made material into a human to replace natural organs or tissues—have promise to be able to extend the quality, quantity, and functionality of life.

- Ketamine Therapy – Ketamine is the only legal psychedelic medicine available in the United States that can be administered by physicians for treating depression, PTSD, suicidal inclinations and mental issues not considered clinical-level psychopathology. In my practice, those who have used Ketamine report improved cognitive performance, greater emotional control, and rediscovery of their purposes and selves. Ketamine can enhance feelings of calm, acceptance, and openness, which can help patients come to terms with challenging life circumstances, both past and present. Ketamine integrative treatment can lead to epiphanic moments and helps foster confidence in overcoming previously insurmountable life obstacles. Ketamine creates opportunities for identifying and transforming ingrained patterns of thought, emotion, and behavior. With integration guidance, clients can apply these garnered insights and rewire responses to traumatic events, life challenges, and daily choices, finding new opportunities for transformation where previously barriers stood in the way. Ketamine also increases BDNF, which promotes the formation of new neurons (neurogenesis) and neuronal connections (synaptogenesis).

Ketamine therapy can be used alone or in combination with intravenous infusion therapy depending on the condition(s) being addressed. Techniques from neurolinguistic programming and neuroassociative conditioning may also be applied. This multi-modality approach serves to remove any emotional and mental blocks that are otherwise taking up cognitive bandwidth. Clients suffering from a range of mood disorders, chronic pain syndromes, migraines, and other chronic health conditions have experienced favorable outcomes.

Think of the mind like a computer's operating system. Occasionally, bad apps are accidentally downloaded, or computer viruses may invade—these could come from the form of childhood or adult traumas, disempowering beliefs/subconscious programs, or negative thought loops. These faulty apps and viruses will slow your operating system and negatively affect all applications of the computer, which is the equivalent of how negative thought patterns or mindsets can lead to poor emotional and physiologic states. A reboot or a visit to the computer repair shop may be needed to get the computer running like new again. For select clients, Ketamine therapy may allow access to clear some negative programming in order to achieve an elevated BioEnergetic state.

These are just some of the modalities available in longevity centers worldwide. However, in my concierge practice, these scientific break-throughs share the front seat with the more holistic elements I've outlined in this book.

With this book, my aim was to give you and those you serve the tools necessary to become your own best medicine. I know that if you implement the Bioenergetic Model on your own, into your everyday life, you will see transformational results not only in you, but all those around you.

For additional information on my concierge practice or our corporate offerings (including keynotes, workshops, and consulting), please visit kienvuu.com.

Thank you again for investing in YOU. Remember always... YOU are your best Medicine.